Teen Health Series

Accident and Safety Information for Teens, Second Edition

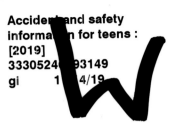

Accident and Safety Information for Teens, Second Edition

Health Tips about Medical Emergencies, Traumatic Injuries, and Emergency Preparedness

Including Facts about Motor Vehicle Accidents, Burns, Poisoning, Firearms, Natural Disasters, National Security Threats, and More

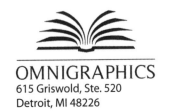

OMNIGRAPHICS
615 Griswold, Ste. 520
Detroit, MI 48226

Table of Contents

Part Three: Motor Vehicle Safety

Part Four: Safety at Home, School, and Work

Part Five: Outdoor and Recreation Safety

Part Six: Emergency and Disaster Preparedness

Part Seven: If You Need More Information

Preface

About This Book

According to statistics compiled by the National Center for Statistics and Analysis (NCSA), accidents are the leading cause of death among children and youth between the ages of 0 to 19 years. In 2016, 6.5 percent of the U.S. population represents young people of the age group 15 to 19. About 2,433 teens of age group 16 to 19 were killed as the result of motor vehicle injury, or teens between age group 16 to 19 died every day through motorcycle crashes and more than 100 were injured. In the age group 0 to 19 years, about 12,000 people died from unintentional injuries, such as traffic accidents, nontraffic-related motor vehicle accidents, poisonings, drownings, falls, exposures to fire and smoke, and violence.

Accident and Safety Information for Teens, Second Edition provides adolescent readers with facts about what to do when accidents happen: when to call 911, what first aid steps can be taken, what to expect in the emergency department or hospital, and how to cope with the aftereffects of a traumatic experience. It describes serious injuries and medical emergencies, including major bleeding, burns, spinal cord injuries, brain injury, drug overdose, and alcohol poisoning. The book also provides information about motor vehicle safety; safety at home, school, and work; and outdoor and recreation-related safety. A separate section discusses emergency and disaster preparedness, including how to make a disaster plan, how to prepare for natural disasters, what steps to take to prepare for national security emergencies, about how people can protect themselves from terrorism of all types. The book concludes with directories of resources for additional help and information.

How to Use This Book

This book is divided into parts and chapters. Parts focus on broad areas of interest; chapters are devoted to single topics within a part.

Part One: Unintentional Injury and Violence: Overview discusses teen death and injury due to violence and accidents, gives statistical information about fatal and nonfatal injuries, describes your brain on an emergency and how to cope up with traumatic experience, gives basic information on first aid and what people should know about 911, and concludes with a report on injury-related emergency department visits.

Part Two: Medical Emergencies and Traumatic Injuries explains complications, prevention, and treatment for animal bites, stings, and insect bites, bleeding, and burns. This part deals with the risk factors, prevention, and diagnosis of fractures and traumatic brain injury and also contains information about spinal cord injury. It concludes with the risk factors, signs, and symptoms of alcohol and opioid overdose.

Part Three: Motor Vehicle Safety describes the leading cause of death for U.S. teens and traffic safety. It describes the development of safe driving skills, the proper use of safety belts and airbags, appropriate care for tires and headlights, and the special challenges related to driving during inclement weather. Problems associated with driving in, drowsy, drunk, and drugged states, speeding, and aggressive driving are discussed, along with what one should do after a car accident. The part concludes with chapters that address the special concerns of motorcyclists and pedestrians.

Part Four: Safety at Home, School, and Work discusses the safety that teens should be aware of at home, school, and workplace. The chapters explain fire, gardening, electrical and power outage safety, and the dangers of carbon monoxide. The part concludes with the safety measures that a working teen should know.

Part Five: Outdoor and Recreation Safety describes sports injury prevention tips and offers suggestions for avoiding dangers and being safe while bicycling, swimming, boating, driving all-terrain vehicles, snowmobiling, skating, skateboarding, skiing, and snowboarding.

Part Six: Emergency and Disaster Preparedness describes the process of planning ahead for natural disasters and national security emergencies. It offers information about how to build a kit for disaster management and what to expect in the event of a tornado, hurricane, flood, winter storm, thunderstorm, lightning, or other incidents associated with the untamed aspects of nature. It also explains steps that can be taken to be ready to respond to human-made disasters, such as chemical accidents and acts of terrorism and bioterrorism.

Part Seven: If You Need More Information includes directories of resources for additional facts about first aid, medical emergencies, and disaster preparedness.

Bibliographic Note

This volume contains documents and excerpts from publications issued by the following U.S. government agencies: Agricultural Research Service (ARS); Centers for Disease Control and Prevention (CDC); *Eunice Kennedy Shriver* National Institute of Child Health and Human Development (NICHD); Federal Bureau of Investigation (FBI); Federal Emergency

Management Agency (FEMA); Health Resources and Services Administration (HRSA); National Highway Traffic Safety Administration (NHTSA); National Institute of Arthritis and Musculoskeletal and Skin Diseases (NIAMS); National Institute of General Medical Sciences (NIGMS); National Institute of Mental Health (NIMH); National Institute on Alcohol Abuse and Alcoholism (NIAAA); National Institute on Drug Abuse (NIDA); National Institutes of Health (NIH); National Transportation Safety Board (NTSB); National Weather Service (NWS); Occupational Safety and Health Administration (OSHA); Office of Disease Prevention and Health Promotion (ODPHP); Office on Women's Health (OWH); U.S. Consumer Product Safety Commission (CPSC); U.S. Department of Homeland Security (DHS); U.S. Department of Transportation (DOT); U.S. Fire Administration (USFA); and U.S. General Services Administration (GSA).

It may also contain original material produced by Omnigraphics and reviewed by medical consultants.

The photograph on the front cover is © Voyagerix/Shutterstock.

Medical Review

Omnigraphics contracts with a team of qualified, senior medical professionals who serve as medical consultants for the *Teen Health Series*. As necessary, medical consultants review reprinted and originally written material for currency and accuracy. Citations including the phrase "Reviewed (month, year)" indicate material reviewed by this team. Medical consultation services are provided to the *Teen Health Series* editors by:

Dr. Vijayalakshmi, MBBS, DGO, MD
Dr. Senthil Selvan, MBBS, DCH, MD
Dr. K. Sivanandham, MBBS, DCH, MS (Research), PhD

About The *Teen Health Series*

At the request of librarians serving today's young adults, the *Teen Health Series* was developed as a specially focused set of volumes within Omnigraphics' *Health Reference Series*. Each volume deals comprehensively with a topic selected according to the needs and interests of people in middle school and high school. Teens seeking preventive guidance, information about disease warning signs, medical statistics, and risk factors for health problems will find answers to their questions in the *Teen Health Series*. The Series, however, is not intended to serve as a tool for diagnosing illness, in prescribing treatments, or as a substitute for the physician/patient relationship. All people concerned about medical symptoms or the possibility of disease are encouraged to seek professional care from an appropriate healthcare provider.

If there is a topic you would like to see addressed in a future volume of the *Teen Health Series*, please write to:

Editor
Teen Health Series
Omnigraphics
615 Griswold, Ste. 520
Detroit, MI 48226

A Note About Spelling And Style

Teen Health Series editors use *Stedman's Medical Dictionary* as an authority for questions related to the spelling of medical terms and the *Chicago Manual of Style* for questions related to grammatical structures, punctuation, and other editorial concerns. Consistent adherence is not always possible, however, because the individual volumes within the Series include many documents from a wide variety of different producers and copyright holders, and the editor's primary goal is to present material from each source as accurately as is possible following the terms specified by each document's producer. This sometimes means that information in different chapters may follow other guidelines and alternate spelling authorities. For example, occasionally a copyright holder may require that eponymous terms be shown in possessive forms (Crohn's disease vs. Crohn disease) or that British spelling norms be retained (leukaemia vs. leukemia).

Part One
Unintentional Injury and
Violence: Overview

Chapter 1

Teen Injury and Death: The Plagues of Accident and Violence

Injuries and violence are widespread in society. Both unintentional injuries and those caused by acts of violence are among the top 15 killers for Americans of all ages. Many people accept them as "accidents," "acts of fate," or as a "part of life." However, most events resulting in injury, disability, or death are predictable and preventable.

Health Impact of Injury and Violence

Unintentional injuries and violence-related injuries can be caused by a number of events, such as motor vehicle crashes and physical assault, and can occur virtually anywhere. No matter what the circumstances of the event are, injuries can have serious, painful, and debilitating physical and emotional health consequences, many of which are long term or permanent, including:

- Hospitalization
- Brain injury
- Poor mental health
- Disability
- Premature death

While their extent, severity, and impact may vary, injuries from any cause can significantly influence the physical, mental, and economic well-being of individuals, families, and communities nationwide.

(Source: "Injury and Violence," HealthyPeople.gov, Office of Disease Prevention and Health Promotion (ODPHP).)

About This Chapter: Text in this chapter begins with excerpts from "Injury and Violence Prevention," HealthyPeople.gov, Office of Disease Prevention and Health Promotion (ODPHP), December 7, 2010. Reviewed July 2019; Text beginning with the heading "Injury and Violence across the Life Stages" is excerpted from "Injury and Violence," HealthyPeople. gov, Office of Disease Prevention and Health Promotion (ODPHP), October 31, 2011. Reviewed July 2019.

Why Are Injury and Violence Prevention Important?

Injuries are the leading cause of death for Americans between the ages of 1 and 44, and the leading cause of disability for all ages, regardless of sex, race/ethnicity, or socioeconomic status. More than 180,000 people die from injuries each year, and approximately 1 in 10 individuals sustains a nonfatal injury serious enough to be treated in a hospital emergency department.

Beyond their immediate health consequences, injuries and violence have a significant impact on the well-being of Americans by contributing to:

- Premature death
- Years of potential life lost
- Disability and disability-adjusted life years lost
- Poor mental health
- High medical costs
- Lost productivity

The effects of injuries and violence extend beyond the injured person or victim of violence to family members, friends, co-workers, employers, and communities.

Injury and Violence across the Life Stages

Injury and violence are pressing public-health concerns at every stage of life. While older adults and children are most vulnerable to sustaining an injury that requires medical attention, Americans of all ages are susceptible to injury and violence.

Children

Injuries resulting from motor vehicle accidents are the leading cause of death for children between the ages of 0 and 19. Each year, approximately 2.8 million children go to the hospital emergency department for injuries caused by falling.

Suffocation is the leading cause of injury death for infants 1 year of age and younger, and drowning for children between the ages of 1 and 4.

A history of exposure to adverse experiences in childhood, including exposure to violence and maltreatment, is associated with health risk behaviors, such as smoking, alcohol and drug use, and risky sexual behavior, as well as with obesity, diabetes, sexually-transmitted diseases (STDs), attempted suicide, and other health problems.

Adolescents and Young Adults

Approximately 72 percent of all deaths among adolescents between the ages of 10 and 24 are attributed to injuries from 4 causes: motor vehicle crashes (30%), all other unintentional injuries (15%), homicide (15%), and suicide (12%).

More than 1 million serious sports-related injuries occur each year among adolescents between the ages of 10 and 17.

Determinants of Injury and Violence

An individual's risk of injury and violence may be impacted by many social, personal, economic, and environmental factors. For example, the physical environment, both in the home and community, can affect the rate of injuries related to falls, fires, burns, road traffic incidents, drowning, and violence.

Understanding these various determinants of health and how they may overlap to create disparities in injury and violence is key to improving the health and safety of all Americans. For example:

- Communities and streets can be designed to reduce pedestrian, bicyclist, and motor vehicle-related injuries.

- Exercise programs, medication reviews, home modifications, and regular vision screening can prevent falls among older adults.

- Housing, economic development, and education initiatives show promise in reducing rates of crime and violence.

Chapter 2

Statistics for Fatal and Nonfatal Injury

Unintentional injuries—such as those caused by burns, drowning, falls, poisoning, and road traffic accidents—are the leading cause of morbidity and mortality among children in the United States. Each year, among those between 0 and 19 years of age, more than 12,000 people die from unintentional injuries, and more than 9.2 million are treated in emergency departments for nonfatal injuries.

The Centers for Disease Control and Prevention's (CDC) *Patterns of Unintentional Injuries among 0 to 19-Year-Olds in the United States, 2000 to 2006* uses data from the National Vital Statistics Systems (NVSS) and the National Electronic Injury Surveillance System (NEISS)—All Injury Program to provide an overview of unintentional injuries related to drowning, falls, fires or burns, poisoning, suffocation, and transportation-related injuries, among others, during the period 2000 to 2006. Results are presented by age and sex, as well as the geographic distribution of injury death rates by state.

> The total lifetime medical and work loss costs of injuries and violence in the United States was $671 billion in 2013. The costs associated with fatal injuries was $214 billion while nonfatal injuries accounted for over $457 billion.
>
> Injuries, including all causes of unintentional and violence-related injuries combined, account for 59 percent of all deaths among people ages 1 to 44 years of age in the United States.
>
> *(Source: "Cost of Injuries and Violence in the United States," Centers for Disease Control and Prevention (CDC).)*

About This Chapter: This chapter includes text excerpted from "CDC Childhood Injury Report," Centers for Disease Control and Prevention (CDC), December 23, 2015. Reviewed July 2019.

Injury Deaths

On average, 12,175 children between 0 and 19 years of age died each year in the United States from an unintentional injury.

Males had higher injury death rates than females. The death rate for males was almost two times the rate for females, and males had a higher injury death rate compared to females in all childhood age groups.

Injuries due to transportation were the leading cause of death for children.

- The highest death rates were among occupants of motor vehicles in traffic.

- There were also a substantial number of pedestrian and cyclist deaths among children.

Combining all unintentional injury deaths among those between 0 and 19 years of age, traffic-related motor vehicle deaths were the leading cause.

The leading causes of injury death differed by age group.

- For children less than one year of age, two-thirds of injury deaths were due to suffocation.

- Drowning was the leading cause of injury death for those between one and four years of age.

- For children between 5 and 19 years of age, most injury deaths were due to being an occupant in a motor vehicle during a traffic crash.

Risk for injury death varied by race.

- Injury death rates were highest for American Indian and Alaska Natives and were lowest for Asian or Pacific Islanders.

- Overall death rates for Whites and African Americans were approximately the same.

Injury death rates varied by state depending upon the cause of death. Overall, states with the lowest injury death rates were in the northeast. Fire and burn death rates were highest in some of the southern states.

Death rates from transportation-related injuries were highest in some southern states and some states of the upper plains, while lowest rates occurred in states in the northeast region.

For injury causes with an overall low burden, death rates greatly varied by age. The poisoning death rate for those older than 15 years of age was at least 5 times the rates of the younger age groups, and the suffocation death rate for infants was over 16 times the rates for all older age groups.

Nonfatal Injuries

An estimated 9.2 million children annually had an initial emergency department visit for an unintentional injury. Males generally had higher nonfatal injury rates than females. For children between 1 and 19 years of age, nonfatal injury rates were higher among males than females, while the rates were approximately the same for those under 1 year.

Injuries due to falls were the leading cause of nonfatal injury.

- Each year, approximately 2.8 million children had an initial emergency department visit for injuries from a fall.

- For children less than 1 year of age, falls accounted for over 50 percent of nonfatal injuries.

The majority of nonfatal injuries are from five causes.

- Falls were the leading cause of nonfatal injury for all groups less than 15 years of age.

- For children between 0 and 9 years of age, the next 2 leading causes were being struck by or against an object and animal bites or insect stings.

- For children between 10 and 14 years of age, the next leading causes were being struck by or against an object and overexertion.

- For children between 15 and 19 years of age, the 3 leading causes of nonfatal injuries were being struck by or against an object, falls, and motor vehicle occupant injuries.

Nonfatal injury rates varied by age group.

- Nonfatal suffocation rates were highest for those less than 1 year of age.

- Rates for fires or burns and drowning were highest for children 4 years of age and younger.

- Children between 1 and 4 years of age had the highest rates of nonfatal falls and poisoning.

- Injury rates related to motor vehicles was highest in children between 15 and 19 years of age.

Chapter 3

Youth Violence and Its Consequences

What Is Youth Violence?

Youth violence is the intentional use of physical force or power to threaten or harm others that is committed by young people between the ages of 10 and 24. Youth violence typically involves young people hurting peers who are unrelated to them and who they may or may not know well. Youth violence can take different forms. Examples include fights, bullying, threats involving weapons, and gang-related violence. A young person can be involved with youth violence as a victim, offender, or witness.

Youth violence starts early. Physical aggression can be common among toddlers, but most children learn alternatives to using violence to solve problems and express their emotions before starting school. Some children may remain aggressive and become more violent. Some early-childhood risk factors include impulsive behavior, poor emotional control, and lack of social and problem-solving skills. Many risk factors are the result of experiencing chronic stress, which can alter and/or harm the brain development of children and youth.

Youth violence is an adverse childhood experience and is connected to other forms of violence, including child abuse and neglect, teen dating violence, adult intimate-partner violence, sexual violence, and suicide. Different forms of violence have common risk and protective factors, and victims of one form of violence are more likely to experience other forms of violence.

About This Chapter: This chapter includes text excerpted from "Preventing Youth Violence," Centers for Disease Control and Prevention (CDC), February 26, 2019.

How Big Is the Problem of Youth Violence?

Thousands of people experience youth violence every day. While the magnitude and types of youth violence vary across communities and demographic groups, youth violence negatively impacts youth in all communities—urban, suburban, rural, and tribal.

Youth violence is common. Nearly one in five high-school students reported being bullied on school property in the last year, and about one in seven were electronically bullied (via texting, Instagram, Facebook, or other social media).

Youth violence kills and injures. Homicide is the third leading cause of death for young people between the ages of 10 and 24. Each day, about 14 young people are victims of homicide and about 1,300 are treated in emergency departments for nonfatal assault-related injuries.

Youth violence is costly. Youth homicides and nonfatal physical assault-related injuries result in more than $21 billion annually in combined medical and lost productivity costs alone, not including costs associated with the criminal justice system; psychological and social consequences for victims, perpetrators, and their families; or costs incurred by communities.

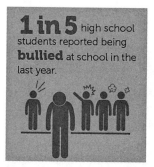
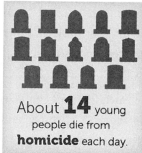
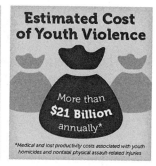

Figure 3.1. Problems of Youth Violence

What Are the Consequences of Youth Violence?

Youth violence has serious and lasting effects on the physical, mental, and social health of young people. It is a leading cause of death for young people and results in more than 475,000 nonfatal injuries each year. The impact of youth violence goes beyond physical consequences. Adverse childhood experiences, such as youth violence, are associated with negative health and well-being outcomes across the life course. Youth violence increases the risk for behavioral and mental-health difficulties, including future violence perpetration and victimization, smoking, substance use, obesity, high-risk sexual behavior, depression, academic difficulties, school dropout, and suicide.

Youth violence affects entire communities. Violence increases healthcare costs, decreases property value, and disrupts social services. Youth violence negatively impacts perceived and actual safety, participation in community events, youth school attendance, and the viability of businesses. Addressing the short- and long-term consequences of violence strains community resources and limits the resources that states and communities have to address other needs and goals.

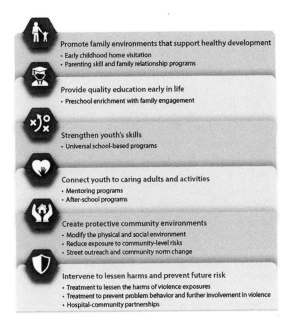

Figure 3.2. How You Can Stop Youth Violence before It Starts

STRYVE Action Council

The STRYVE Action Council is a multisector consortium of organizations that works at the national level to advance youth violence prevention efforts in states and communities.

The Action Council's work in support of state and local efforts includes:

- Increasing awareness that youth violence is a preventable public-health issue.
- Expanding the network of national, state, and local organizations involved in youth-violence prevention.
- Informing national, state, and local policy that advances youth-violence prevention strategies.

(Source: "Partnerships to Prevent Youth Violence," Centers for Disease Control and Prevention (CDC).)

Chapter 4

This Is Your Brain on Emergencies

There is a fire in your building. Your plane is about to crash. A woman beside you on the street suddenly collapses.

What do you do?

Well, that depends. Every one of us is at risk for these kinds of unexpected intrusions into our day-to-day lives. What you do about it depends on whether or not you are prepared—not just physically, but also mentally.

In any situation, some things are likely to be out of your control: the size of the fire, who is flying the plane, what is wrong with the injured person. Some things, however, are up to you. Being aware of how you might react can go a long way toward making a bad situation better.

Know Yourself

In a crisis, your brain wants to make decisions, and these decisions are not always the best ones. The good news is that there are steps you can take to be a better decision-maker in emergencies. There is science behind the way people react to stressful situations, and we can use it to our advantage.

Science tells us that people behave in high-stress incidents in certain ways. What you do largely depends on what your stress level is. If your heart rate soars above 175 beats per minute, you are more likely to go into shutdown mode and not be able to think clearly or act.

About This Chapter: This chapter includes text excerpted from "This Is Your Brain on Emergencies," Centers for Disease Control and Prevention (CDC), December 12, 2016.

A technique called "combat breathing" (inhale through your nose, hold, exhale through your mouth, hold) has been shown to reduce your heart rate by 20 to 30 beats per minute. Controlling your emotion and stress level will help as you go through the decision-making process.

Deep Breathing

Deep breathing is a good way to relax. Most of us breathe from the chest, which is known as "shallow breathing." When you breathe deeply, your body takes in more oxygen. You exhale more carbon dioxide. Your body naturally "resets" itself to a more relaxed and calm state. Deep breathing can be useful for anyone who has stress. You can practice deep breathing during your workday when you're feeling stressed or anxious. And you can choose to take a couple minutes and breathe deeply each day, or just use it when you need it. Deep breathing doesn't just work for handling day-to-day stress. Symptoms such as anxiety, "panic" or feeling "stuck in alarm mode" often respond well to deep breathing.

(Source: "Relaxation Exercise: Deep Breathing," U.S. Department of Veterans Affairs (VA).)

During the decision-making process, your mind will most likely move through three stages:

- Denial

- Deliberation

- Decisive action

Knowing these stages—and preparing for them ahead of time—can help you recognize and deal with what is going on around you more effectively.

Denial: This Is Not Happening

Have you ever heard gunfire in your neighborhood and blamed it on a firecracker? That is denial, and it is perfectly normal. You do not want to believe bad things are happening. You do not want to panic or look silly.

In emergencies, you often look to people around you for cues about what you should do. (Is everyone else running and screaming, or are they sitting quietly in their chairs? Are others stopping to help?) This is known as "social proof." Social proof is a psychological phenomenon that happens whenever people are not sure what to do. You assume others around you to know more about the situation, and so you do what they do, whether it is the right thing or not.

You also know that a person is less likely to take responsibility when others are present. You assume that other people are responsible for taking action or that they have already done so.

This is called "diffusion of responsibility," and it means you are actually more likely to get help when you are with a single person than when you are in a large group of people.

All are susceptible to believing these things, which make it easy to deny that an emergency is really happening or that all need to do something about it.

Deliberation: What Are My Options?

Once you have recognized the emergency, you will begin to consider your options. If you are smart, you have already started this process before the emergency happens. Maybe you participated in a fire drill at work, or you counted exactly how many rows there are between you and the emergency exit on the plane, or you took a first aid class in your community. The more you have prepared, the more options you will have to work with.

One thing you can do to prepare everywhere you go is called "scripting." All it requires is a little bit of imagination. Pay attention to your surroundings and see what is available to you. Check for exits (and consider windows as possible exits). Be nosy, especially when it concerns your safety. Then, run different scenarios in your head. Where would you go if you had to get out? Who would you call if you need help? What will you do if there is a fire? A robbery? A bomb threat? Think about the possibilities ahead of time.

Everybody hates the idea that we practice for emergency events. But it is practice, and practice helps you understand what to do or how to react when you do not have a lot of time. Not only can practice save your life, but if you know how to save yourself, emergency responders on the scene can use their time and effort to save others. You are one less person who needs saving, and that saves lives.

Decisive Action: It Is Go Time

You have acknowledged there is a problem. You have considered your options. The next step is to take decisive action. With all the information you have, what are you going to do next?

Before you take action:

- Calm yourself.

- Shift your emotion. If you do get mad, use that anger as energy.

- Stay fit—if you are more fit, you are likely to be more rational.

Now is the time to put your plans into motion. Go to the exit, call for help, take cover, give cardiopulmonary resuscitation (CPR), or do whatever you have decided to do.

In most crisis situations, there is no definite right or wrong. There is no perfect way—only the best we can do. The most important thing is to do something. In almost every case, an imperfect plan is better than no plan, and action is better than inaction.

Remember, if you depend on everyone else to take care of you, you are leaving the most important person out. Do not wait to make a plan. Know yourself, know your situation, and be prepared to save your own life.

Chapter 5

What You Should Know about 911

An emergency is any situation that requires immediate assistance from the police, the fire department, or an ambulance. Examples include:

- A fire

- A crime, especially if it is in progress

- A car crash, especially if someone is injured

- A medical emergency, especially for symptoms that require immediate medical attention

If you are not sure whether the situation is a true emergency, officials recommend calling 911 and letting the call taker determine whether you need emergency help.

> The 911 system was designed to provide a universal, easy-to-remember number for people to reach police, fire, or emergency medical assistance from any phone in any location, without having to look up specific phone numbers.
>
> Today, people communicate in ways that the designers of the original 911 system could not have envisioned: wireless phones, text and video messages, social media, Internet Protocol (IP)-enabled devices, and more.
>
> *(Source: "About the National 911 Program," National 911 Program, National Highway Traffic Safety Administration (NHTSA).)*

About This Chapter: Text in this chapter begins with excerpts from "Need to Call or Text 911," National 911 Program, National Highway Traffic Safety Administration (NHTSA), July 2, 2010. Reviewed July 2019; Text under the heading "Using 911 Appropriately" is excerpted from "Using 911 Appropriately," National 911 Program, National Highway Traffic Safety Administration (NHTSA), November 18, 2017; Text under the heading "Frequently Asked Questions" is excerpted from "Frequently Asked Questions," National 911 Program, National Highway Traffic Safety Administration (NHTSA), December 14, 2015. Reviewed July 2019.

Using 911 Appropriately

Generally speaking, people are aware that they should call 911 in an emergency, but they are less aware of the circumstances in which they should not call 911. The result is that many requests to 911 do not involve true emergencies, which overloads the 911 system with nonemergency calls.

Most people rarely face emergency situations and lack firsthand experience with 911. They may have unrealistic expectations about what will happen when they contact 911 for emergency assistance.

There is a growing need for targeted and well-coordinated public education efforts about how to use 911 appropriately. Because 911 system capabilities vary across the nation, the National 911 Program supports local efforts to promote public awareness and the effective use of 911 resources.

If you dial 911 by mistake, or if a child in your home dials 911 when no emergency exists, do not hang up—that could make officials think that an emergency exists, and possibly send responders to your location. Instead, simply explain to the call taker what happened.

Frequently Asked Questions
What Happens When You Call 911?

Many 911 call centers follow protocols that guide callers through a sequence of questions to quickly obtain information necessary for dispatching the right responders to the right location. Call takers may also provide instructions about what to do until help arrives. Even though protocols are designed to help call takers reassure callers and take charge of the situation, the experience can be stressful for a 911 caller who is not accustomed to dealing with emergencies. When you call 911, be prepared to answer the call taker's questions, which may include:

- The location of the emergency, including the street address

- The phone number you are calling from

- The nature of the emergency

- Details about the emergency, such as a physical description of a person who may have committed a crime, a description of any fire that may be burning, or a description of injuries or symptoms being experienced by a person having a medical emergency

Remember, the call taker's questions are important to get the right kind of help to you as quickly as possible. Be prepared to follow any instructions the call taker gives you. Many 911 centers can tell you exactly what to do until help arrives, such as providing step-by-step instructions to aid someone who is choking or needs first aid or CPR. Do not hang up until the call taker instructs you to do so.

Can I Text 911 for Emergency Assistance?

Access to 911 through text messaging is significantly limited across the United States, although efforts are underway to accept text messages at call centers nationwide. If you need emergency assistance, it is always best to call 911 from a landline or wireless phone.

Even if text-to-911 services are available in your market, a voice call remains the best way to reach 911. If you send a text message to 911, and text-to-911 services are not available in your community, you should receive a bounceback message from the wireless provider telling you that the message was not delivered.

What Should I Do If I Accidentally Dial 911?

If you dial 911 by mistake, or if a child in your home dials 911 when no emergency exists, do not hang up—that could make 911 officials think that an emergency exists, and possibly send responders to your location. Instead, simply explain to the call taker what happened.

Can I Dial 911 from a Wireless Phone without a Wireless Calling Plan?

All wireless phones, even those that are not subscribed to or supported by a specific carrier, can be used to dial 911. These uninitialized phones are often used to place malicious or fake calls to 911 call centers. These calls are a burden on the 911 system because they require the answering center to confirm whether or not an emergency truly exists.

How Do I Place a "Test" Call to Make Sure 911 Works for Me?

Test calls confirm that your local 911 service can receive your 911 call and has the correct location information. Test calls can be scheduled by contacting your local 911 call center via its nonemergency phone number.

To find the nonemergency, 10-digit phone number for your local 911 call center, conduct an Internet search for the nonemergency number of the local law enforcement agency (LEA).

When you speak with law enforcement staff, explain that you do not have an emergency, but would like to request the local 911 call center's nonemergency 10-digit number.

How Do I Know My Local 911 Has the Correct Address for My Home or Business?

When calling 911, it is important to know your location and be able to provide 911 with the correct address and closest cross streets or landmarks. If you would like to contact your local 911 call center to confirm the address that correlates with your phone number is correct, do not dial 911. Rather, contact your local public safety answering point (PSAP) or call center through its nonemergency, 10-digit phone number.

To locate this number, conduct an Internet search for the nonemergency number of the local law enforcement agency. When you speak with law enforcement staff, explain that you do not have an emergency, but would like to request the local 911 call center's nonemergency 10-digit number.

How Can I Reach 911 in a Different State, County, or City?

With a few exceptions, 911 calls cannot be transferred to other jurisdictions except between call centers within a county and between adjacent counties. The best option to obtain emergency assistance in a different state, county, or city is to dial the 10-digit phone number for law enforcement in the community where assistance is needed. Those numbers can be found on the local law enforcement agency's websites.

For corporations interested in providing emergency assistance support to clients nationwide, a list of 911 call center 10-digit emergency phone numbers can be obtained by contacting the National Emergency Number Association (NENA).

How Can I Register My Voice over Internet Protocol Phone for 911?

Voice over Internet Protocol (VoIP) service allows users to place and receive calls to and from traditional phone numbers using an Internet connection and can be used in place of traditional phone service. Because VoIP phones can be used anywhere an Internet connection is available, the 911 call center cannot locate callers unless the VoIP device is registered to a physical address through the VoIP provider. Anytime the VoIP phone is moved from one location to another, the owner should contact the provider to update the new physical location of the device.

What Are 911 Apps?

A number of private companies have developed and sell a variety of smartphone computer applications intended to supplement the use of 911. Because 911 system capabilities vary across the United States, it is important that application developers have confirmed that their company/organization has the legal authority to contact 911 on a caller's behalf. If you have any questions regarding the use of a particular app with the call center in your community, please contact the application provider directly to ask questions about legal authority or the use of their application by a specific 911 call center.

Who Manages 911 Call Centers?

911 professionals are employed by a variety of local and state agencies, including law enforcement agencies, fire departments, emergency-management agencies, and Information Technology (IT) services, either as sworn or civilian personnel.

Are 911 Call Takers Certified?

Some 911 professionals are certified as emergency medical dispatchers (EMDs), emergency fire dispatchers (EFDs) or emergency police dispatchers (EPDs), which means they have received additional specialized training to assist callers in all types of emergencies. Managers and supervisors may also be certified as emergency-number professionals, or ENPs, demonstrating that they have mastered the comprehensive knowledge base necessary to manage an emergency-number program.

Why Are 911 Fees Included on My Landline or Wireless Bill?

Local governments pass laws that allow them to collect 911 fees through your local telephone service or wireless provider. The fees collected are distributed to help pay for emergency communication and response services in your area. Enhanced 911 (E911), which enables a wireless device to transmit its phone number and geographic location to the 911 call center, is an example of how wireless services have upgraded their delivery of 911 calls over time. According to the Federal Communications Commission (FCC), some wireless service providers may choose to pass their costs of providing E911 service on to their customers and this charge may also be described as an E911 charge on your wireless telephone bill.

What Is 911 Fund Diversion?

Revenues collected for 911 are sometimes diverted to other purposes by states or local governments. The Federal Communications Commission (FCC) is charged with monitoring and reporting on states' collection and usage of 911 funds, including information regarding the diversion of 911 funds from their intended purposes.

Chapter 6

First Aid Basics

Get Medical Attention for All Injuries

It is very important for you to get immediate treatment for every injury, regardless how small you may think it is. Many cases have been reported where a small and seemingly unimportant injury, such as a splinter wound or a puncture wound, quickly led to an infection, threatening the health and limb of the injured person. Even the smallest scratch is large enough for dangerous germs to enter, and in large bruises or deep cuts, germs come in by the millions.

Control Bleeding with Pressure

Bleeding is the most visible result of an injury. Each of us has between five and six quarts of blood in our body. Most people can lose a small amount of blood with no problem, but if a quart or more is quickly lost, it could lead to shock and/or death.

- One of the best ways to treat bleeding is to place a clean cloth on the wound and apply pressure with the palm of your hand until the bleeding stops.

- Elevate the wound above the victim's heart, if possible, to slow down the bleeding at the wound site.

- Apply pressure to the nearest supplying blood vessel (major pressure point) located either on the inside of the upper arm between the shoulder and elbow, or in the groin area where the leg joins the body.

About This Chapter: This chapter includes text excerpted from "First Aid Basics," Agricultural Research Service (ARS), U.S. Department of Agriculture (USDA), December 8, 2016.

Direct pressure is better than a pressure point or a tourniquet (a device, such as a bandage twisted tight with a stick, to control the flow of blood) because direct pressure stops blood circulation only at the wound.

Once the bleeding stops, do not try to remove the cloth that is against the open wound as it could disturb the blood clotting and restart the bleeding. Only use the pressure points if elevation and direct pressure have not controlled the bleeding.

Never use a tourniquet except in response to an extreme emergency, such as a severed arm or leg. Tourniquets can damage nerves and blood vessels, and they can cause the victim to lose an arm or leg.

Treat Physical Shock Quickly

Shock can threaten the life of the victim of an injury if it is not treated quickly. Even if the injury does not directly cause death, the victim can go into shock and die. Shock occurs when the body's important functions are threatened by not getting enough blood or when the major organs and tissues do not receive enough oxygen. Some of the symptoms of shock are a pale or blue-ish skin color that is cold to the touch, vomiting, dull and sunken eyes, and unusual thirst.

Shock requires medical treatment to be reversed, so all you can do is prevent it from getting worse.

- Generally, keep the victim lying flat on the back.
- Maintain an open airway for breathing.
- Control any obvious bleeding, and elevate the legs about 12 inches unless an injury makes it impossible.
- Prevent the loss of body heat by covering the victim (over and under) with blankets.
- Do not give the victim anything to eat or drink because this may cause vomiting.

A victim who is unconscious or bleeding from the mouth should lie on one side so breathing is easier. Stay with the victim until medical help arrives.

Move the Injured Person Only When Absolutely Necessary

Never move an injured person unless fire or explosives are involved. The major concern with moving an injured person is making the injury worse, which is especially true with spinal cord injuries (SCIs).

If you must move an injured person, try to drag her or him by the clothing around the neck or shoulder area. If possible, drag the person onto a blanket or large cloth and then drag the blanket.

Perform the Heimlich Maneuver on Choking Victims

Ask the victim to cough, speak, or breathe. If the victim can do none of these things:

- Stand behind the victim and locate the bottom rib with your hand.

- Move your hand across the abdomen to the area above the navel then make a fist and place your thumb side on the stomach.

- Place your other hand over your fist and press into the victim's stomach with a quick upward thrust until the food is dislodged.

Flush Burns Immediately with Water

There are a many different types of burns. They can be thermal burns, chemical burns, electrical burns, or contact burns. Each of the burns can occur in a different way, but treatment for them is very similar.

For thermal, chemical, or contact burns, the first step is to run cold water over the burn for a minimum of 30 minutes. If the burn is small enough, keep it completely under water. Do not use ice.

- Flushing the burn takes priority over calling for help. Flush the burn first.

- If the victim's clothing is stuck to the burn, do not try to remove it. Remove clothing that is not stuck to the burn by cutting or tearing it.

- Cover the burn with a clean, cotton material. If you do not have clean, cotton material, do not cover the burn with anything.

Do not scrub the burn and do not apply any soap, ointment, or home remedies. Also, do not offer the burn victim anything to drink or eat, but keep the victim covered with a blanket to maintain a normal body temperature until medical help arrives.

Electrical burn treatment is a little different. Do not touch a victim who has been in contact with electricity unless you are clear of the power source. If the victim is still in contact with the power source, electricity will travel through the victim's body and electrify you when you reach to touch them. Once the victim is clear of the power source, your priority is:

- Check for any airway obstruction, and check breathing and circulation. Administer cardiopulmonary resuscitation (CPR) if necessary.

- Once the victim is stable, begin to run cold water over the burns for a minimum of 30 minutes.

- Do not move the victim, and do not scrub the burns or apply any soap, ointment, or home remedies.

- After flushing the burn, apply a clean, cotton cloth to the burn. If cotton is not available, do not use anything. Keep the victim warm and still, and try to maintain a normal body temperature until medical help arrives.

Use Cool Treatment for Heat Exhaustion or Stroke

Heat exhaustion and heat stroke are two different things, although they are commonly confused as the same condition.

Heat exhaustion can occur anywhere there is poor air circulation, such as around an open furnace or heavy machinery, or even if the person is poorly adjusted to very warm temperatures. The body reacts by increasing the heart rate and strengthening blood circulation. Simple heat exhaustion can occur due to loss of body fluids and salts. The symptoms are usually excessive fatigue, dizziness, and disorientation accompanied by a normal skin temperature but a damp and clammy feeling.

To treat heat exhaustion, move the victim to a cool spot and encourage drinking of cool water and rest.

Heat stroke is much more serious and occurs when the body's sweat glands shut down. Some symptoms of heat stroke are mental confusion; collapsing into unconsciousness; and a fever accompanied by dry, mottled skin. A heat stroke victim will die quickly, so do not wait for medical help to arrive; assist immediately.

The first thing you can do is move the victim to a cool place out of the sun and begin pouring cool water over the victim. Fan the victim to provide good air circulation until medical help arrives.

Respond Appropriately to Poisoning

The first thing to do is get the victim away from the poison. Then, provide treatment appropriate to the form of the poisoning.

Pills or any other solid form. Remove it from the victim's mouth using a clean cloth wrapped around your finger. Do not try this with infants because it could force the poison further down their throat.

Gas. You may need a respirator to protect yourself. After checking the area first for your safety, remove the victim from the area and take them to fresh air.

Corrosive to the skin. Remove the clothing from the affected area and flush with water for 30 minutes. Take the poison container or label with you when you call for medical help because you will need to be able to answer questions about the poison. Try to stay calm and follow the instructions you are given. If the poison is in contact with the eyes, flush the victim's eyes for a minimum of 15 minutes with clean water.

First Aid to Heart Attack

Symptoms include chest pains; difficulty breathing; nausea; sweating; and a weak, rapid pulse. If you suspect a person has suffered a heart attack, search for an identification card or bracelet for additional steps or a doctor's telephone number. Question eyewitnesses about what has occurred. First aid for a heart attack is as follows:

- Place the victim in a comfortable position.

- Raise the head and chest if breathing is difficult.

- If breathing stops, apply artificial respiration by physician or person trained in CPR.

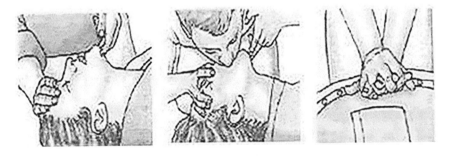

Figure 6.1. First Aid for a Person Suspected of Heart Attack

If the pulse becomes absent, give CPR if trained and retrieve the facility's automated external defibrillator (AED) unit.

- Tip the individual's head to open the airway. Look, listen, and feel for breathing.

- Restore breathing. Give mouth-to-mouth artificial respiration.

- Restore circulation. Check carotid pulse. If absent, apply external cardiac compression on the victim's breast bone.

  - 15 chest compression at 80 to 100 per minute, alternate with 2 slow full lung inflations, then repeat 15 compressions.

Use an AED, and only use chest compression when instructed by the AED unit during in-between shock sessions.

Keep a First Aid Kit Checklist

In order to administer effective first aid, it is important to maintain adequate supplies in each first aid kit. First aid kits can be purchased commercially and are already stocked with the necessary supplies, or one can be made by including the following items:

- **Adhesive bandages** are available in a large range of sizes for minor cuts, abrasions, and puncture wounds

- **Butterfly closures** hold wound edges firmly together.

- **Rolled gauze** allows freedom of movement and is recommended for securing the dressing and/or pads. These are especially good for hard-to-bandage wounds.

- **Nonstick sterile pads** are soft, super absorbent pads that provide a good environment for wound healing. Rolled gauze is recommended for bleeding and draining wounds, burns, infections.

- **First aid tapes** of various types should be included in each kit. These include adhesive, which is waterproof and extra strong for times when rigid strapping is needed; clear, which stretches with the body's movement and are good for visible wounds; cloth, recommended for most first aid taping needs, including taping heavy dressings (less irritating than adhesive); paper, which is recommended for sensitive skin and is used for light and frequently changed dressings.

Items that also can be included in each kit are tweezers, first aid cream, a thermometer, an analgesic or equivalent, and an ice pack.

Report All Work-Related Injuries to Your Superiors

As with getting medical attention for all injuries, it is equally important that you report all work-related injuries to your superior.

Taking Action Right Away Can Save a Life

Take these steps now so you'll be ready in an emergency:

- Know when to call 911.
- Learn how to help someone who is choking or hurt.
- Take a class to learn first aid, CPR (cardiopulmonary resuscitation), and AED (automated external defibrillator).
- Keep a first aid kit at home and in your car.

Remember, it is important to plan ahead and be prepared for injuries and emergencies. Simple actions can save lives.

(Source: "Learn First Aid," Office of Disease Prevention and Health Promotion (ODPHP), U.S. Department of Health and Human Services (HHS).)

Chapter 7

Injury-Related Emergency Department Visits: A Report

Data from the National Hospital Ambulatory Medical Care Survey, 2009 to 2010

Injury is the leading cause of death and a major source of morbidity among children and adolescents in the United States. The emergency department (ED) plays an important role in the care of injuries, and these visits often represent the initial contact with a provider for the injury. This report examines nationally representative data on injury-related ED visits by children and adolescents 18 years of age and younger in the United States during 2009 to 2010. Injury-related ED visit rates were also compared for the age groups 0 to 4, 5 to 12, and 13 to 18 years of age, as these correspond to the preschool, school-age, and teen life periods, respectively.

- In 2009 to 2010, an annual average of 11.9 million injury-related ED visits were made by children and adolescents 18 years of age and younger in the United States.

- The injury-related ED visit rate was 151 per 1,000 persons 18 years of age and younger, and rates were higher for males than for females for all age groups (0 to 4 years, 5 to 12 years, and 13 to 18 years).

- The injury-related ED visit rates among persons 5 to 12 years of age and 13 to 18 years of age were higher for non-Hispanic Black persons than for other race and ethnicity groups.

- Leading causes of injury-related ED visits among both males and females included falls and striking against or being struck unintentionally by objects or persons. Visit rates were higher for males than for females for both of these causes.

About This Chapter: This chapter includes text excerpted from "Injury-Related Emergency Department Visits by Children and Adolescents: United States, 2009–2010," Centers for Disease Control and Prevention (CDC), November 6, 2015. Reviewed July 2019.

Injury-Related Emergency Department Visit Rates for Children and Adolescents

- In 2009 to 2010, there were an estimated 33.7 million annual average ED visits by persons 18 years of age and younger in the United States, and 11.9 million (35.3%) of these visits were injury related.

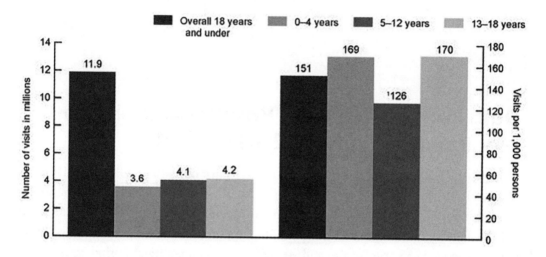

Figure 7.1. Number and Rate of Injury-Related Emergency Department Visits for Persons Aged 18 Years and Under: United States, 2009 to 2010 *(Source: Centers for Disease Control and Prevention (CDC)/National Center for Health Statistics (NCHS), National Hospital Ambulatory Medical Care Survey (NHAMCS), 2009–2010.)*

[1] *Visit rate is significantly different (p < 0.05) than for other age groups, based on a two-tailed t test.*

Notes: *Figures are based on 2-year averages. A sample of 6,185 injury-related emergency department visits were made by patients aged 18 years and under, representing an annual average weighted total of 11.9 million injury-related visits. Visit rates are based on July 1, 2009, and July 1, 2010, set of estimates of the civilian non-institutionalized population of the United States, as developed by the Population Division, U.S. Census Bureau.*

- The annual average ED visit rate was 151 per 1,000 persons 18 years of age and younger.

- A "u-shaped" curve was observed for the injury-related ED visit rates by children and adolescents, which was lowest in the 5 to 12-year age group compared with the 0 to 4 and 13 to 18-year age groups.

Did the Injury-Related Emergency Department Visit Rates for Children and Adolescents Vary by Sex?

- In 2009 to 2010, the injury-related ED visit rate was higher among males than females in all age groups.

- Among both males and females, the visit rate was lowest in the 5 to 12-year age group compared with the 0 to 4 and 13 to 18-year age groups.

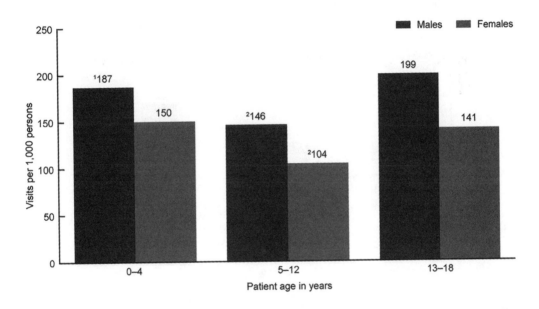

Figure 7.2. Injury-Related Emergency Department Visit Rates by Sex for Persons Aged 18 Years and Under: United States, 2009 to 2010 *(Source: Centers for Disease Control and Prevention (CDC)/National Center for Health Statistics (NCHS), National Hospital Ambulatory Medical Care Survey (NHAMCS), 2009–2010.)*

[1] Visit rate is significantly different (p < 0.05) for males than for females in all age groups, based on a two-tailed t test.

[2] Visit rate is significantly different (p < 0.05) than for other age groups, based on a two-tailed t test.

Notes: *Figures are based on 2-year averages. Visit rates are based on July 1, 2009, and July 1, 2010, set of estimates of the civilian noninstitutionalized population of the United States, as developed by the Population Division, U.S. Census Bureau.*

Did the Injury-Related Emergency Department Visit Rates for Children and Adolescents Vary by Race and Ethnicity?

- In both the 5 to 12 and 13 to 18-year age groups, the injury-related ED visit rate was highest among non-Hispanic Black persons, followed by non-Hispanic White persons, and Hispanic persons.

- In the 0 to 4-year age group, the injury-related ED visit rate was higher among non-Hispanic Black persons compared with Hispanic persons. The observed difference between non-Hispanic Black persons and non-Hispanic White persons did not reach statistical significance.

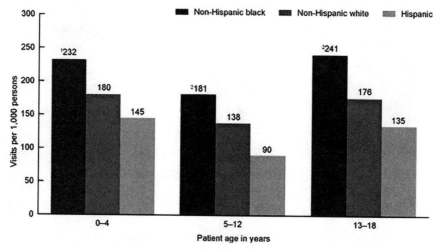

Figure 7.3. Injury-Related Emergency Department Visit Rates by Race and Ethnicity for Persons Aged 18 Years and Under: United States, 2009 to 2010 *(Source: Centers for Disease Control and Prevention (CDC)/National Center for Health Statistics (NCHS), National Hospital Ambulatory Medical Care Survey (NHAMCS), 2009–2010.)*

[1] *Visit rates within the 0–4 age group are significantly different (p < 0.05) for non-Hispanic Black persons compared with Hispanic persons based on two-tailed t tests. The difference between non-Hispanic Black persons and non-Hispanic White persons did not reach statistical significance.*

[2] *Visit rates within the 5–12 and 13–18 year age groups are significantly different (p < 0.05) for all race and ethnicity groups shown based on two-tailed t tests.*

Notes: *Figures are based on 2-year averages. Visit rates are based on July 1, 2009, and July 1, 2010, set of estimates of the civilian noninstitutionalized population of the United States, as developed by the Population Division, U.S. Census Bureau.*

What Were the Leading Causes of Injury-Related Emergency Department Visits among Children and Adolescents, and Did Visit Rates for These Causes Vary by Sex?

- Leading causes of injury-related ED visits among both males and females 18 years of age and younger included falls and striking against or being struck unintentionally by objects or persons.

- Injury-related ED visit rates were higher for males than for females 18 years of age and younger for unintentional injuries caused by falls, striking against or being struck by objects or persons, and cutting or piercing instruments or objects.

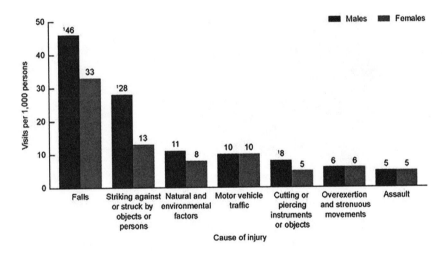

Figure 7.4. Emergency Department Visit Rates for Leading Causes of Injury by Sex for Persons Aged 18 Years and Under: United States, 2009 to 2010 *(Source: Centers for Disease Control and Prevention (CDC)/National Center for Health Statistics (NCHS), National Hospital Ambulatory Medical Care Survey (NHAMCS), 2009–2010.)*

[1] Visit rate is significantly different (p < 0.05) for males than for females based on a two-tailed t test.

Notes: *Based on "Supplementary Classification of External Cause of Injury and Poisoning" in the International Classification of Diseases, Ninth Revision, Clinical Modification (ICD–9–CM). Causes shown are unintentional with the exception of assault. Figures are based on 2-year averages. Visit rates are based on the July 1, 2009, and July 1, 2010, set of estimates of the civilian noninstitutionalized population of the United States, as developed by the Population Division, U.S. Census Bureau.*

What Were the Primary Expected Sources of Payment for Injury-Related Emergency Department Visits by Children and Adolescents?

- The most frequently recorded primary expected sources of payment for injury-related ED visits by children and adolescents were Medicaid or Children's Health Insurance Program (CHIP) (41.7%) and private insurance (40.7%).

- Injury-related ED visits by children and adolescents with no insurance comprised 8.6 percent of visits.

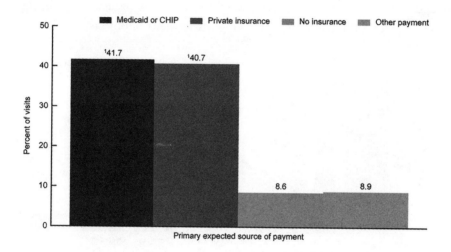

Figure 7.5. Percentage of Injury-Related Emergency Department Visits by Primary Expected Source of Payment for Persons Aged 18 Years and Under: United States, 2009 to 2010 (Source: Centers for Disease Control and Prevention (CDC)/National Center for Health Statistics (NCHS), National Hospital Ambulatory Medical Care Survey (NHAMCS), 2009–2010.)

[1] Percentages are significantly different (p < 0.05) for Medicaid or Children's Health Insurance Program (CHIP) and private insurance compared with no insurance or other payment based on two-tailed t tests.

Notes: The following payment types were used for this analysis: Medicaid or CHIP; private insurance; no insurance, which includes self-pay and no charge or charity; and other, which includes Medicare, workers' compensation, categories not otherwise listed, unknown, and blank. Figures are based on two-year averages. Numbers may not add to totals because of rounding.

Child and adolescent injuries represent a serious public-health problem in the United States. Over one-third of ED visits made by persons 18 years of age and younger—an average of 11.9 million visits annually—were injury related in 2009 to 2010. The annual average injury-related ED visit rate was 151 per 1,000 persons 18 years of age and younger. A number of findings related to injury-related ED visits during that time period were identified. The injury-related ED visit rate was lower in the 5 to 12-year age group compared with the 0 to 4 and 13 to 18-year age groups, and the rate was higher among males compared with females in each age group. Among persons aged 5 to 12 and 13 to 18 years, the injury-related ED visit rate was highest among non-Hispanic Black persons compared with other race and ethnicity groups analyzed. Leading causes of injury-related ED visits among both males and females 18 years of age and younger included falls and striking against or being struck unintentionally by objects or persons. Males had higher visit rates for unintentional injuries caused by falls, striking against or being struck by objects or persons, and cutting or piercing instruments or objects.

Injury-prevention objectives covering a broad range of issues have recently been outlined for Healthy People 2020 with the goal of preventing injury and violence and reducing their consequences. The National Hospital Ambulatory Medical Care Survey (NHAMCS) data are used to track the injury-prevention objectives related to reducing ED visits for nonfatal injuries overall and for nonfatal traumatic brain injuries (TBIs). Monitoring and evaluating data related to child and adolescent injuries will remain important for informing injury-prevention efforts in this population.

Chapter 8

Coping with a Traumatic Experience

A traumatic event is a shocking, scary, or dangerous experience that affects someone emotionally. These situations may be natural, such as a tornado or earthquake. They can also be caused by other people, such as a car accident, crime, or terror attack.

How individuals respond to traumatic events is an important area of research for the National Institute of Mental Health (NIMH). Researchers are exploring the factors that help people cope, as well as the factors that increase their risk for problems following the event.

Common Responses to a Traumatic Event

A person's response to a traumatic event may vary. Responses include feelings of fear, grief, and depression. Physical and behavioral responses include nausea, dizziness, and changes in appetite and sleep pattern as well as withdrawal from daily activities. Responses to trauma can last for weeks to months before people start to feel normal again. Most people report feeling better within three months after a traumatic event. If the problems become worse or last longer than one month after the event, the person may be suffering from posttraumatic stress disorder (PTSD).

(Source: "Coping with a Traumatic Event," Centers for Disease Control and Prevention (CDC).)

About This Chapter: This chapter includes text excerpted from "Coping with Traumatic Events," National Institute of Mental Health (NIMH), February 2017.

Warning Signs

There are many different responses to potentially traumatic events. Most people have intense responses immediately following and often for several weeks or even months after a traumatic event. These responses can include:

- Feeling anxious, sad, or angry

- Trouble concentrating and sleeping

- Continually thinking about what happened

For most people, these are normal and expected responses, and they generally lessen with time. Healthy ways of coping in this time period include avoiding alcohol and other drugs; spending time with loved ones and trusted friends who are supportive; and trying to maintain normal routines for meals, exercise, and sleep. In general, staying active is a good way to cope with stressful feelings.

However, in some cases, stressful thoughts and feelings after a trauma continue for a long time and interfere with everyday life. For people who continue to feel the effects of the trauma, it is important to seek professional help. Some signs that an individual may need help include:

- Worrying a lot or feeling very anxious, sad, or fearful

- Crying often

- Having trouble thinking clearly

- Having frightening thoughts, reliving the experience

- Feeling angry

- Having nightmares or difficulty sleeping

- Avoiding places or people that bring back disturbing memories and responses

Physical responses to trauma may also mean that an individual needs help. Physical symptoms may include:

- Headaches

- Stomach pain and digestive issues

- Feeling tired

- Racing heart and sweating

- Being very jumpy and easily startled

Those who already had mental-health problems or who have had traumatic experiences in the past, those who are faced with ongoing stress, or those who lack support from friends and family may be more likely to develop stronger symptoms and need additional help. Some people turn to alcohol or other drugs to cope with their symptoms. Although substance use can temporarily cover up symptoms, it can also make life more difficult.

Mental-health problems can be treated. If you or someone you know needs help, talk with your healthcare provider.

What Can You Do for Yourself?

There are many things you can do to cope with traumatic events. Understand that your symptoms may be normal, especially right after the trauma.

Keep to your usual routine. Take the time to resolve day-to-day conflicts so they do not add to your stress.

Do not shy away from situations, people and places that remind you of the trauma. Find ways to relax and be kind to yourself. Turn to family, friends, and clergy person for support, and talk about your experiences and feelings with them. Participate in leisure and recreational activities.

Recognize that you cannot control everything.

Recognize the need for trained help, and call a local mental-health center.

(Source: "Coping with a Traumatic Event," Centers for Disease Control and Prevention (CDC).)

Part Two
Medical Emergencies and Traumatic Injuries

Chapter 9

Animal Bites

Cat Bites and Scratches

Cat-scratch disease (CSD) is a bacterial infection spread by cats. The disease spreads when an infected cat licks a person's open wound or bites or scratches a person hard enough to break the surface of the skin. About 3 to 14 days after the skin is broken, a mild infection can occur at the site of the scratch or bite. The infected area may appear swollen and red with round, raised lesions, and it can have pus. The infection can feel warm or painful. A person with CSD may also have a fever, headache, poor appetite, and exhaustion. Later, the person's lymph nodes closest to the original scratch or bite can become swollen, tender, or painful.

Wash cat bites and scratches well with soap and running water. Do not allow cats to lick your wounds. Contact your doctor if you develop any symptoms of cat-scratch disease or infection.

Cat-scratch disease is caused by a bacterium called "*Bartonella henselae.*" About 40 percent of cats carry *B. henselae* at some time in their lives, although most cats with this infection show no signs of illness. Kittens younger than one year of age are more likely to have *B. henselae* infection and to spread the germ to people. Kittens are also more likely to scratch and bite while they play and learn how to attack prey.

About This Chapter: Text under the heading "Cat Bite and Scratches" is excerpted from "Cat-Scratch Disease," Centers for Disease Control and Prevention (CDC), April 30, 2014. Reviewed July 2019; Text under the heading "Dog Bites" is excerpted from "Preventing Dog Bites," Centers for Disease Control and Prevention (CDC), April 8, 2019; Text under the heading "Snakebite" is excerpted from "How to Prevent or Respond to a Snake Bite," Centers for Disease Control and Prevention (CDC), September 21, 2018.

How Cats and People Become Infected

Cats can get infected with *B. henselae* from flea bites and flea dirt (droppings) getting into their wounds. By scratching and biting at the fleas, cats pick up the infected flea dirt under their nails and between their teeth. Cats can also become infected by fighting with other cats that are infected. The germ spreads to people when infected cats bite or scratch a person hard enough to break their skin. The germ can also spread when infected cats lick at wounds or scabs that you may have.

Serious but Rare Complications

Although rare, CSD can cause people to have serious complications. CSD can affect the brain, eyes, heart, or other internal organs. These rare complications, which may require intensive treatment, are more likely to occur in children younger than five years of age and people with weakened immune systems.

Prevention

Do:

- Wash cat bites and scratches right away with soap and running water.

- Wash your hands with soap and running water after playing with your cat, especially if you live with young children or people with weakened immune systems.

- Since cats less than one year of age are more likely to have CSD and spread it to people, persons with a weakened immune system should adopt cats older than one year of age.

Do not:

- Play rough with your pets because they may scratch and bite

- Allow cats to lick your open wounds

- Pet or touch stray or feral cats

Available Tests and Treatment

Talk to your doctor about testing and treatments for CSD. People are only tested for CSD when the disease is severe and the doctor suspects CSD based on the patient's symptoms. CSD is typically not treated in otherwise healthy people.

Dog Bites

Dog bites can cause pain and injury, but they can also spread germs that cause infection. Nearly one in five people bitten by a dog requires medical attention. Any dog can bite—know how to enjoy dogs without getting bitten.

Dogs can be our closest companions; in the United States, over 36 percent of households own at least 1 dog. Dogs have been proven to decrease stress, increase our exercise levels, and are playmates for children. But sometimes, man's best friend will bite. In addition to causing pain, injury, or nerve damage, dog bites can become infected, putting the bite victim at risk for illness or in rare cases death.

Although the idea of being bitten by a dog is scary, it does not mean you need to avoid dogs completely. If you work or live around dogs, be aware of the risks and learn how to enjoy being around dogs without getting bitten.

Know the Risks

Children are more likely to be bitten by a dog than adults, and when they are, the injuries can be more severe. Over half of dog bite injuries occur at home with dogs that are familiar to us. Having a dog in the household is linked to a higher likelihood of being bitten than not having a dog. As the number of dogs in the home increases, so does the likelihood of being bitten. Adults with two or more dogs in the household are five times more likely to be bitten than those living without dogs at home. Among adults, men are more likely than women to be bitten by a dog.

How to Prevent Dog Bites

Do:

- Always ask if it is okay to pet someone else's dog before reaching out to pet the dog.

- When approached by an unfamiliar dog, remain motionless ("be still like a tree").

- If a dog knocks you over, curl into a ball with your head tucked and your hands over your ears and neck.

- Immediately let an adult know about any stray dogs or dogs that are behaving strangely.

Do not:

- Approach an unfamiliar dog

- Run from a dog

- Panic or make loud noises

- Disturb a dog that is sleeping, eating, or caring for puppies

- Pet a dog without allowing it to see and sniff you first

- Encourage your dog to play aggressively

- Let small children play with a dog unsupervised

What to Do If an Unfamiliar Dog Approaches You and You Do Not Want to Interact with It

- Stay still, and be calm.

- Do not panic or make loud noises.

- Avoid direct eye contact with the dog.

- Say "No" or "Go Home" in a firm, deep voice.

- Stand with the side of your body facing the dog. Facing a dog directly can appear aggressive to the dog. Instead, keep your body turned partially or completely to the side.

- Slowly raise your hands to your neck, with your elbows in.

- Wait for the dog to pass or slowly back away.

What to Do If You Are Bitten or Attacked by a Dog
Protect Yourself

- Put your purse, bag, or jacket between you and the dog.

- If you are knocked down, curl into a ball with your head tucked in and your hands over your ears and neck.

Wash Wounds with Soap and Water

When you get to a safe place, immediately wash wounds with soap and water. Seek medical attention, especially:

- For minor wounds:

  - Wash the wound thoroughly with soap and water.

- Apply an antibiotic cream.

- Cover the wound with a clean bandage.

- See a healthcare provider if the wound becomes red, painful, warm, or swollen; if you develop a fever; or if the dog that bit you was acting strangely.

- For deep wounds:

  - Apply pressure with a clean, dry cloth to stop the bleeding.

  - If you cannot stop the bleeding or you feel faint or weak, call 911 or your local emergency medical services immediately.

  - See a healthcare provider as soon as possible.

- See a healthcare provider:

  - If the wound is serious (uncontrolled bleeding, loss of function, extreme pain, muscle or bone exposure, etc.)

  - If the wound becomes red, painful, warm, or swollen, or if you develop a fever

  - If you do not know if the dog has been vaccinated against rabies

  - If it has been more than five years since your last tetanus shot, and the bite is deep

Report the Bite

- Because anyone who is bitten by a dog is at risk of getting rabies, consider contacting your local animal-control agency or police department to report the incident, especially:

  - If you do not know if the dog has been vaccinated against rabies

  - If the dog appears sick or is acting strangely

- If possible, contact the owner and ensure the animal has a current rabies vaccination. You will need the rabies vaccine license number; name of the veterinarian who administered the vaccine; and the owner's name, address, and phone number.

Diseases You Can Get from Dog Bites

In addition to causing injury, dog bites can spread germs from dogs to people. Up to 18 percent of dog bites become infected with bacteria. Over 60 different kinds of bacteria have been found in dog mouths, but only a handful of these germs can make you sick. Dog bites can cause the following diseases:

- Rabies is one of the most serious diseases people can get from dog bites. Although getting rabies from a dog in the United States is rare, it is still a risk. The Rabies is a virus that affects the brain and is almost always fatal once symptoms appear. Rabies virus is most commonly spread through the bite and saliva of an infected animal. The disease can be prevented by vaccinating dogs. People who are bitten by a dog should speak with a healthcare provider to see if rabies vaccination is necessary.

- *Capnocytophaga* bacteria live in the mouths of people, dogs, and cats. These bacteria do not make dogs or cats sick. Rarely, *Capnocytophaga* can spread to people through bites, scratches, or close contact from a dog or cat and cause illness. Most people who have contact with dogs or cats do not become sick, but people with a weakened immune system are at a greater risk of becoming sick because it is harder for their bodies to fight infections.

- Pasteurella is a type of bacteria seen in over half of infected dog bite wounds. Pasteurella commonly causes a painful, red infection at the site of the bite, but it can cause a more serious disease in people with weakened immune systems. There may also be swollen glands, swelling in the joints, and difficulty moving.

- Methicillin-resistant *Staphylococcus aureus* (MRSA) is a type of staph infection that is resistant to a certain group of antibiotics. Dogs and other animals can carry MRSA without showing any symptoms, but the bacteria can cause skin, lung, and urinary tract infections (UTIs) in people. In some people, MRSA can spread to the bloodstream or lungs and cause life-threatening infections.

- Tetanus is a toxin produced by a type of bacteria called "*Clostridium tetani.*" This toxin causes rigid paralysis in people and could be a problem in deep bite wounds.

Any dog can bite, but if you understand the risks for dog bites and know how to protect yourself, you will reduce your likelihood of getting sick or injured.

Snakebite

After a natural disaster, snakes may have been forced from their natural habitats and moved into areas where they would not normally be seen or expected. When you return to your home, be cautious of snakes that may have sought shelter in your home. If you see a snake in your home, immediately call the animal-control agency in your county.

How to Prevent Snakebite

- Be aware of snakes that may be swimming in the water to get to higher ground and those that may be hiding under debris or other objects.

- If you see a snake, back away from it slowly and do not touch it.

Signs of Snakebite

If you have to walk in high water, you may feel a bite but not know that you were bitten by a snake. You may think it is another kind of bite or scratch. Pay attention to the following snakebite signs.

Depending on the type of snake, the signs and symptoms may include:

- A pair of puncture marks at the wound

- Redness and swelling around the bite

- Severe pain at the site of the bite

- Nausea and vomiting

- Labored breathing (in extreme cases, breathing may stop altogether)

- Disturbed vision

- Increased salivation and sweating

- Numbness or tingling around your face and/or limbs

What to Do If You or Someone Else Is Bitten by a Snake

- If you or someone you know are bitten, try to see and remember the color and shape of the snake, which can help with treatment of the snakebite.

- Keep the bitten person still and calm. This can slow down the spread of venom if the snake is venomous.

- Seek medical attention as soon as possible.

- Dial 911, or call local emergency medical services (EMS).

- Apply first aid if you cannot get the person to the hospital right away.

- Lay or sit the person down with the bite below the level of the heart.

- Tell her or him to stay calm and still.

- Wash the wound with warm soapy water immediately.

- Cover the bite with a clean, dry dressing.

What Not to Do If You or Someone Else Is Bitten by a Snake

- Do not pick up the snake or try to trap it (this may put you or someone else at risk for a bite).

- Do not apply a tourniquet.

- Do not slash the wound with a knife.

- Do not suck out the venom.

- Do not apply ice or immerse the wound in water.

- Do not drink alcohol as a painkiller.

- Do not drink caffeinated beverages.

How to Prevent Animal Bites and Complications from Bites

Animal bites rarely are life-threatening, but if they become infected, you can develop serious medical problems.

To prevent animal bites and complications from bites:

- Never pet, handle, or feed unknown animals
- Leave snakes alone
- Watch your children closely around animals
- Vaccinate your cats, ferrets, and dogs against rabies
- Spay or neuter your dog to make it less aggressive
- Get a tetanus booster if you have not had one recently
- Wear boots and long pants when you are in areas with venomous snakes

If an animal bites you, clean the wound with soap and water as soon as possible. Get medical attention if necessary.

(Source: "Animal Bites," MedlinePlus.gov, National Institutes of Health (NIH).)

Chapter 10

Stings and Biting Insects

Stinging or biting insects or scorpions can be hazardous. Stinging or biting insects include bees, wasps, hornets, and fire ants.

The health effects of stinging or biting insects or scorpions range from mild discomfort or pain to a lethal reaction for those who are allergic to the insect's venom. Anaphylactic shock is the body's severe allergic reaction to a bite or sting, and it requires immediate emergency care. Thousands of people are stung by insects each year, and as many as 90 to 100 people in the United States die as a result of allergic reactions. This number may be underreported as deaths may be mistakenly diagnosed as heart attacks or sunstrokes or may be attributed to other causes.

It is important for everyone to train themselves about their risk of exposure to insects and scorpions, how they can prevent and protect themselves from stings and bites, and what they should do if they are stung or bitten.

Bees, Wasps, and Hornets

Bees, wasps, and hornets are most abundant in the warmer months. Nests and hives may be found in trees under roof eaves; or on equipment, such as ladders. They are found throughout the United States.

About This Chapter: This chapter includes text excerpted from "Insects and Scorpions," Centers for Disease Control and Prevention (CDC), May 31, 2018.

Recommendations

You should protect yourself from stinging insects by learning about:

- Your risk of exposure

- Insect identification

- How to prevent exposure

- What to do if stung

You should take the following steps to prevent insect stings:

- Wear light-colored, smooth-finished clothing.

- Avoid perfumed soaps, shampoos, and deodorants.

- Do not wear cologne or perfume.

- Avoid bananas and banana-scented toiletries.

- Wear clean clothing and bathe daily. (Sweat may anger bees.)

- Wear clothing to cover as much of the body as possible.

- Avoid flowering plants when possible.

- Keep work areas clean. Social wasps thrive in places where humans discard food.

- Remain calm and still if a single stinging insect is flying around. (Swatting at an insect may cause it to sting.)

- If you are attacked by several stinging insects at once, run to get away from them. (Bees release a chemical when they sting, which may attract other bees.)

- Go indoors.

- A shaded area is better than an open area to get away from the insects.

- If you are able to physically move out of the area, do not attempt to jump into water. Some insects (particularly Africanized honey bees) are known to hover above the water, continuing to sting once you surface for air.

- If a bee comes inside your vehicle, stop the car slowly, and open all the windows.

- If you are a person with a history of severe allergic reactions to insect bites or stings, you should consider carrying an epinephrine auto-injector (EpiPen) and wearing a medical identification bracelet or necklace stating your allergy.

First Aid

If you are stung by a bee, wasp, or hornet:

- Have someone stay with you to be sure that you do not have an allergic reaction.

- Wash the site with soap and water.

- Remove the stinger using gauze wiped over the area or by scraping a fingernail over the area.

- Never squeeze the stinger or use tweezers.

- Apply ice to reduce swelling.

- Do not scratch the sting as this may increase swelling, itching, and the risk of infection.

Fire Ants

Imported fire ants first came to the United States around 1930. Now there are five times more ants per acre in the United States than in their native South America. The fire ants that came to the United States escaped their natural enemies and thrived in the southern landscape.

Fire ants bite and sting. They are aggressive when stinging and inject venom, which causes a burning sensation. Red bumps form at the sting, and within a day or two, they become white fluid-filled pustules.

Fire ants are found mostly in the southeastern United States, with limited geographic distribution in New Mexico, Arizona, and California.

Recommendations

You should learn about:

- Your risk of exposure

- How to identify fire ants and their nests

- How to prevent exposure

- What to do if you are bitten or stung

You should take the following steps to prevent fire ant stings and bites:

- Do not disturb or stand on or near ant mounds.

- Be careful when lifting items (including animal carcasses) off the ground, as they may be covered in ants.

- Fire ants may also be found on trees or in water, so always look over the area before starting to work.

First Aid

If you are a person with a history of severe allergic reactions to insect bites or stings, you should consider carrying an epinephrine auto-injector and wearing a medical identification bracelet or necklace stating your allergy.

You should take the following steps if you are stung or bitten by fire ants:

- Rub off ants briskly, as they will attach to the skin with their jaws.

- Antihistamines may help.

- Follow the directions on the packaging.

- Drowsiness may occur.

- Get someone to take you to an emergency medical facility immediately if a sting causes severe chest pain, nausea, severe sweating, loss of breath, serious swelling, or slurred speech.

Scorpions

Scorpions usually hide during the day and are active at night. They may be hiding under rocks, wood, or anything else lying on the ground. Some species may also burrow into the ground. Most scorpions live in dry, desert areas. However, some species can be found in grasslands, forests, and inside caves. They can be found especially in the southern and southwestern United States.

Symptoms

Symptoms of a scorpion sting may include:

- A stinging or burning sensation at the injection site (very little swelling or inflammation)

- Positive "tap test" (i.e., extreme pain when the sting site is tapped with a finger)

- Restlessness

- Convulsions

- Roving eyes

- Staggering gait

- Thick tongue sensation

- Slurred speech

- Drooling

- Muscle twitches

- Abdominal pain and cramps

- Respiratory depression

These symptoms usually subside within 48 hours, although stings from a bark scorpion can be life-threatening.

Recommendations

You should protect yourself from scorpions by learning about:

- Your risk of exposure

- Scorpion identification

- How to prevent exposure

- What to do if stung

You should take the following steps to prevent scorpion stings:

- Wear long sleeves and pants.

- Wear leather gloves.

- Shake out clothing or shoes before putting them on.

- If you are a person with a history of severe allergic reactions to insect bites or stings, you should consider carrying an epinephrine auto-injector and wearing a medical identification bracelet or necklace stating your allergy.

First Aid

You should take the following steps if you are stung by a scorpion:

- Contact a qualified healthcare provider or poison control center for advice and medical instructions.

- Ice may be applied directly to the sting site (never submerge the affected limb in ice water).

- Remain relaxed and calm.

- Do not take any sedatives.

- Capture the scorpion for identification if it is possible to do so safely.

Anascorp

"Once stung, twice shy" are words to live by in the Southwestern United States, where about 11,000 people a year are stung by scorpions in Arizona alone. Though rarely life threatening, scorpion stings can be extremely painful, causing numbness and burning at the wound site. And there has been little a victim could do to ease the pain. The biologic treatment—called "Anascorp" provides treatment for children and adults and is designed specifically for scorpion stings. Without Anascorp, children experiencing the most severe symptoms usually had to stay in intensive care in the hospital for several days; but when Anascorp was administered, researchers found patients' symptoms disappeared after a few hours in the emergency room—eliminating the need for a hospital stay.

(Source: "Antidote Relieves Scorpion Stings," U.S. Food and Drug Administration (FDA).)

Chapter 11

Bleeding

Bleeding is the loss of blood. It can happen outside or inside the body. You may bleed when you get a cut or other wound. Bleeding can also be due to an injury to internal organs.

Sometimes, bleeding can cause other problems. A bruise is bleeding under the skin. Some strokes are caused by bleeding in the brain. Other bleeding, such as gastrointestinal bleeding, coughing up blood, or vaginal bleeding, can be a symptom of a disease.

Normally, when you bleed, your blood forms clots to stop the bleeding. Severe bleeding may require first aid or a trip to the emergency room. If you have a bleeding disorder, your blood does not form clots normally.

Give First Aid in Case of Emergency

Accidents happen. It is important to know when to call 911 for life-threatening emergencies. While waiting for help to arrive, you may be able to save someone's life. Cardiopulmonary resuscitation (CPR) is for people whose hearts or breathing has stopped, and the Heimlich maneuver is for people who are choking.

You can also learn to handle common injuries and wounds. Cuts and scrapes, for example, should be rinsed with cool water. To stop bleeding, apply firm but gentle pressure, using gauze. If blood soaks through, add more gauze, keeping the first layer in place. Continue to apply pressure.

About This Chapter: Text in this chapter begins with excerpts from "Bleeding," MedlinePlus, National Institutes of Health (NIH), January 25, 2017; Text under the heading "Give First Aid in Case of Emergency" is excerpted from "First Aid," MedlinePlus, National Institutes of Health (NIH), July 13, 2018; Text under the heading "Reach for Emergency Medical Services" is excerpted from "Emergency Medical Services," MedlinePlus, National Institutes of Health (NIH), September 12, 2016.

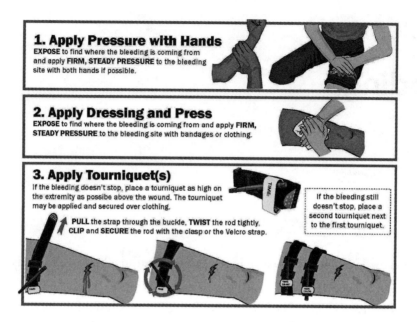

1. Apply Pressure with Hands
EXPOSE to find where the bleeding is coming from and apply **FIRM, STEADY PRESSURE** to the bleeding site with both hands if possible.

2. Apply Dressing and Press
EXPOSE to find where the bleeding is coming from and apply **FIRM, STEADY PRESSURE** to the bleeding site with bandages or clothing.

3. Apply Tourniquet(s)
If the bleeding doesn't stop, place a tourniquet as high on the extremity as possibe above the wound. The tourniquet may be applied and secured over clothing.

PULL the strap through the buckle, **TWIST** the rod tightly, **CLIP** and **SECURE** the rod with the clasp or the Velcro strap.

If the bleeding still doesn't stop, place a second tourniquet next to the first tourniquet.

Figure 11.1. Steps to Stop Bleeding *(Source: "Stop the Bleed," U.S. Department of Homeland Security (DHS).)*

It is important to have a first-aid kit available. Keep one at home and one in your car. It should include a first-aid guide. Read the guide to learn how to use the items, so you are ready in case an emergency happens.

Reach for Emergency Medical Services

If you get very sick or badly hurt and need help right away, you should use emergency medical services. These services use specially trained people and specially equipped facilities.

You may need care in a hospital emergency room (ER). Doctors and nurses there treat emergencies, such as heart attacks and injuries. For some emergencies, you need help where you are. Emergency medical technicians, or EMTs, do specific rescue jobs. They answer emergency calls and give basic medical care. Some EMTs are paramedics—they have training to do medical procedures on site. They usually take you to the ER for more care.

If you or someone you know needs emergency care, go to your hospital's emergency room. If you think the problem is life-threatening, call 911.

Chapter 12

Burns

What Is a Burn?

A burn is tissue damage caused by heat, chemicals, electricity, sunlight, or nuclear radiation. The most common burns are those caused by hot liquid or steam, building fires, and flammable liquids and gases.

Burns are defined by how deep they are and how large an area they cover. A large burn injury is likely to include burned areas of different depths.

Deep burns heal more slowly; are more difficult to treat; and are more prone to complications, such as infections and scarring. Very deep burns are the most life-threatening of all and may require amputation. Types of burns include:

- **First-degree burns** damage the outer layer (epidermis) of the skin. These burns usually heal on their own within a week. A common example is a sunburn.

- **Second-degree burns** damage not only the outer layer but also the layer beneath it (dermis). These burns might need a skin graft—natural or artificial skin to cover and protect the body while it heals—and they may leave a scar.

- **Third-degree burns** damage or completely destroy both layers of skin, including hair follicles and sweat glands, and damage underlying tissues. These burns always require skin grafts.

- **Fourth-degree burns** extend into fat, **fifth-degree burns** into muscle, and **sixth-degree burns** to bone.

About This Chapter: This chapter includes text excerpted from "Burns," National Institute of General Medical Sciences (NIGMS), January 2018.

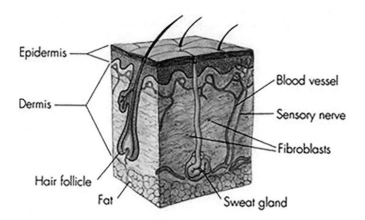

Figure 12.1. Types of Tissues

Cross-section of skin anatomy shows layers and different tissue types.

How Does the Body React to a Severe Burn?

Severe burns cause serious, body-wide problems. At the root of most of these problems is the body's explosive inflammatory response.

A normal inflammatory response protects the body from invaders, such as bacteria, viruses, fungi, cancerous cells, toxins, and foreign materials. It activates in response to infection, injury, or other threats. It is designed to destroy the cause of the problem, contain the damage, and clean up the mess left by dead cells and other debris. But, when faced with large or deep burns, it can overreact, often making the injury more severe and harming the heart, lungs, blood vessels, kidneys, and other organ systems.

During this inflammatory response, there is fluid loss that can cause a sharp and potentially deadly drop in blood pressure that is known as "shock." Fluid can also become trapped inside the body, leading to swelling that is known as "edema." If tissues and organs do not receive enough oxygen because of shock, edema, or something else, they suffer damage and can fail. The lungs, heart, brain, and kidneys are particularly susceptible.

Infection is also a major concern. Burns damage the skin's protective barrier, meaning bacteria and other foreign invaders can sneak in. Burns also weaken the immune system, so the body is less able to fight off threats. Infections can take hold not only in the injured area but also in organs, such as the lungs (pneumonia) and bloodstream (sepsis), where they are potentially lethal.

First Aid for Burns

For minor burns:

- Immerse in fresh, cool water, or apply cool compresses for 10 to 15 minutes.
- Dry the area with a clean cloth. Cover with sterile gauze or a nonadhesive bandage.
- Do not apply ointments or butter; these may cause infection.
- Do not break blisters.
- Over-the-counter (OTC) pain medications may help reduce inflammation and pain.

Call emergency services (911) if:

- Burns cover a large area of the body
- Burns affect the entire thickness of skin
- The victim is an infant or elderly
- The burn was caused by electricity, which can lead to "invisible" burns

(Source: "Burning Issue: Handling Household Burns," NIH News in Health, National Institutes of Health (NIH).)

How Are Burns Treated?

In many cases, healthcare providers cover the burned area using sterile bandages with topical antibiotics (skin creams or ointments) or long-acting, silver-containing dressings to prevent infection.

For third-degree burns and some second-degree ones, patients need extra fluids to maintain blood pressure and prevent shock. Surgeons may treat large burns by removing burned tissue and covering the burn wound with a skin graft. Depending on the severity, location, and nature of a burn, doctors may treat the injury with a combination of natural skin grafts, artificial skin products, and laboratory-grown epidermis.

Injured body parts need to be exercised to maintain their functionality and range of motion.

People with minor burns may be treated at their local hospital. Those with more serious burns might be transferred to a hospital with a special burn unit. Serious burns include any burns that are likely to lead to impaired physical or psychological recovery. The American Burn Association (ABA) maintains an online searchable list of verified burn centers in the United States.

What Is the Prognosis for People Who Have Severe Burns?

A few decades ago, burns covering half the body were often fatal. Now, thanks to research—a large portion of it supported by the National Institute of General Medical Sciences (NIGMS)—people with burns covering 90 percent of their bodies can survive, although they often have permanent impairments and scars.

Chapter 13

Broken Bones and Growth-Plate Injuries

A fracture is a break, and it is usually in a bone. If the broken bone punctures the skin, it is called an "open fracture" or a "compound fracture." Fractures commonly happen because of car accidents, falls, or sports injuries. Other causes are low bone density and osteoporosis, which causes weakening of the bones. Overuse can cause stress fractures, which are very small cracks in the bone.

> Accidental fractures can occur in children who are mobile and active. Household accidents and falls produce the most common accidental fractures: linear skull, clavicle, forearm, and lower leg "toddler's" fractures.
>
> *(Source: "Recognizing When a Child's Injury or Illness Is Caused by Abuse," Office of Juvenile Justice and Delinquency Prevention (OJJDP), U.S. Department of Justice (DOJ).)*

Symptoms of a fracture are:

- Intense pain
- Deformity—the limb looks out of place
- Swelling, bruising, or tenderness around the injury
- Numbness and tingling
- Problems moving a limb

About This Chapter: Text in this chapter begins with excerpts from "Fractures," MedlinePlus, National Institutes of Health (NIH), March 15, 2016; Text under the heading "Growth-Plate Injuries" is excerpted from "Growth Plate Injuries," National Institute of Arthritis and Musculoskeletal and Skin Diseases (NIAMS), May 31, 2014. Reviewed July 2019.

You need to get medical care right away for any fracture. An x-ray can tell if your bone is broken. You may need to wear a cast or splint. Sometimes you need surgery to put in plates, pins, or screws to keep the bone in place.

Growth-Plate Injuries

The growth plate, also known as the "epiphyseal plate" or "physis," is the area of growing tissue near the ends of the long bones in children and adolescents.

Each long bone has at least two growth plates; one at each end. The growth plate determines the future length and shape of the mature bone. Once a child's growth is complete—sometime during adolescence—the growth plates close and are replaced by solid bone.

The growth plates are the weakest areas of a child's growing skeleton. Because they are even weaker than the nearby ligaments and tendons that connect bones to other bones and muscles, growth plates are vulnerable to injury.

Who Gets Growth-Plate Injuries

Growth-plate injuries are more likely to occur:

- In growing children and teens. When a child or teen injures a joint, they are more likely to fracture the growth plate. A similar injury in an adult would cause a sprain.

- Growth-plate fractures occur twice as often in boys as in girls. A girl's body matures at an earlier age than boys. As a result, girls' bones finish growing sooner. When the growth plates finish growing, they are replaced by stronger, solid bone.

- Growth-plate injuries often occur in children and teens who participate in competitive sports or activities such as:

  - Football

  - Basketball

  - Gymnastics

  - Biking

  - Sledding

  - Skiing

  - Skateboarding

Fractures can result from a single traumatic event, such as a fall or automobile accident, or from chronic stress and overuse. Most growth-plate fractures occur in the long bones of the fingers (phalanges) and the outer bone of the forearm (radius). They are also common in the lower bones of the leg (the tibia and fibula).

Types of Growth-Plate Injuries

Depending on the type of damage, the Salter-Harris classification divides most growth-plate fractures into five categories:

- Type I is a fracture through the growth plate and happens when the epiphysis is completely separated from the end of the bone, through the deep layer of the growth plate. The growth plate remains attached to the epiphysis. The doctor may have to put or set the fracture back into place if it is significantly displaced. Type I injuries generally require a cast to protect the plate as it heals. Unless there is damage to the blood supply to the growth plate, the likelihood that the bone will grow normally is excellent.

- Type II is a fracture that runs through the growth plate and metaphysis, but not through the epiphysis. This is the most common type of growth-plate fracture. Type II fractures may need the doctor to set the bones and immobilize the injury. However, this type of injury can heal quickly in younger children, and the doctor may not need to set the bone back into position. If this is the case, the injury heals and strengthens with time.

- Type III fractures run through the growth plate, leading to a separation of epiphysis and growth plate from the metaphysis. This type of injury rarely happens. However, when this type of fracture occurs, it is usually at the lower end the long bones of the lower leg. Surgery is sometimes necessary to restore the joint surface to normal. The outlook or prognosis for growth is good if the blood supply to the separated portion of the epiphysis is still intact and if the joint surface heals in a normal position.

- Type IV fractures run through the growth plate, metaphysis, and epiphysis. Doctors frequent need to perform surgery to restore the joint surface to normal and to perfectly align the growth plate. If perfect alignment is not achieved and maintained during healing, prognosis for growth is poor, and angulation (bending) of the bone may occur. This injury occurs most commonly at the end of the humerus (the upper arm bone) near the elbow.

- Type V is a compression fracture through the growth plate that happens when the end of the bone is crushed, and the growth plate is compressed. This injury is not common.

However, when it happens, it is most likely to occur at the knee or ankle. The prognosis is not as good as the other types of fractures because premature stunting of growth almost always occurs.

- Type VI fractures are included in a newer classification, called the "Peterson classification." This injury happens when a portion of the epiphysis, growth plate, and metaphysis are missing. This usually occurs with open wounds or compound fractures. A type VI growth-plate injury often involves lawn mowers, farm machinery, snowmobiles, or gunshot wounds. All children or teens with a type VI fracture require surgery, and most require additional reconstructive or corrective surgery. Bone growth is almost always stunted.

Symptoms of Growth-Plate Injuries

A child or teen could have symptoms of growth-plate injury when they:

- Complain of persistent pain after a sudden injury
- Limit the amount of time playing after an old injury
- Have changes in the way their limb bends
- Cannot move a limb because of pain
- Have persistent pain after an overuse injury

Whether an injury is acute or due to overuse, a child or teen should see a doctor for evaluation. Some injuries, if left untreated, can lead to permanent damage and interfere with the proper growth of the injured limb.

Causes of Growth-Plate Injuries

Growth-plate injuries happen for many reasons. Most occur after a sudden accident, such as falling or having a hard hit to the limb. The most common causes of growth-plate injuries include:

- Trauma to the limb from a blow or falling down
- Competitive sports (such as football)
- Recreational activities

Sometimes, growth-plate injuries happen when a person overuses a certain part of the body. For example:

- Gymnasts who practice for hours on the uneven bars

- Long-distance runners

- Baseball pitchers perfecting their curveballs

Although many growth-plate injuries are caused by accidents that occur during play or athletic activity, growth plates are also susceptible to other disorders that can alter their normal growth and development. Other possible causes of growth-plate injuries include the following:

- Bone infections

- Child abuse

- Injury from extreme cold (for example, frostbite)

- Radiation and medications

- Neurological disorders

- Genetics

- Metabolic disease

Diagnosis of Growth-Plate Injuries

Doctors diagnose growth-plate injuries by:

- Asking about the injury and how it occurred

- Examining the patient

- Ordering x-rays

Often the doctor will x-ray a child's or teen's injured limb and the opposite limb as well. Because growth plates have not yet hardened into solid bone, neither the structures themselves nor injuries to them show up on x-rays. Instead, growth plates appear as gaps between the metaphysis and the epiphysis. By comparing x-rays of a child's injured limb to those of their noninjured limb, doctors can look for differences that indicate an injury.

Very often the x-ray is negative because the growth-plate line is already there, and the fracture is undisplaced (the two ends of the broken bone are not separated). The doctor can still diagnose a growth-plate fracture on clinical grounds because of the tenderness of the plate. Children do get ligament strains if their growth plates are open, and they often have undisplaced growth-plate fractures.

Other tests doctors may use to diagnose a child's growth-plate injury include:

- Magnetic resonance imaging (MRI)

- Computed tomography (CT)

- Ultrasound

Because these tests enable doctors to see the growth plate and areas of other soft tissue, they can be useful not only in detecting the presence of an injury but also in determining the type and extent of the injury.

Treatment of Growth-Plate Injuries

Treatment for growth-plate injuries depends on the type of injury. In all cases, treatment should be started as soon as possible after injury and will generally involve a mix of the following:

Immobilization

The doctor puts the injured limb in a cast or splint, and the patient is told to limit any activity that puts pressure on the injured area.

Manipulation or Surgery

If the fracture is displaced (meaning the ends of the injured bones no longer meet as they should), the doctor will have to put, or set, the bones or joints back in their correct positions. Doctors do this by:

- **Manipulation.** The doctor uses her or his hands to set the bone.

- **Performing surgery.** Sometimes, the doctor needs to fix the break and hold the growth plate in place with screws or wire. After the procedure, the bone will be set in place (immobilized) so it can heal without moving. This is usually done with a cast that encloses the injured growth plate and the joints on both sides of it.

After manipulation or surgery, the doctor places a cast on the injured area. The cast is left in place until the injury heals, which can take anywhere from a few weeks to two or more months for serious injuries.

The need for manipulation, or surgery, depends on the location and extent of the injury, its effect on nearby nerves and blood vessels, and the child's age.

Strengthening and Range-of-Motion Exercises

The doctor may recommend exercises to strengthen the muscles that support the injured area of the bone. Strengthening can help to improve the patient's ability to move the joint in the way that it should. Doctors usually recommend these after the fracture has healed. A physical therapist can work with a child or teen and her or his doctor to design an appropriate exercise plan. Long-term follow-up is usually necessary to monitor recuperation and growth.

Chapter 14

Spinal Cord Injuries

What Is Spinal Cord Injury?

Spinal cord injury (SCI) is usually associated with what is commonly called a "broken neck" or "broken back." Generally speaking, SCI is damage to the spinal nerves, the body's central and most important nerve bundle, as a result of trauma to the backbone.

Most cases of SCI take place when trauma breaks and squeezes the vertebrae, or the bones of the back. This, in turn, damages the axons—the long nerve cell wires that pass through vertebrae, carrying signals between the brain and the rest of the body. The axons might be crushed or completely severed by this damage. Someone with injury to only a few axons might be able to recover completely from their injury. On the other hand, a person with damage to all axons will most likely be paralyzed in the areas below the injury.

An SCI is described by its level, type, and severity. The level of injury for a person with SCI is the lowest point on the spinal cord below which sensory feeling and motor movement diminish or disappear.

The level is denoted by the letter-and-number name of the vertebra at the injury site (such as C3, T2, or L4).

- There are seven cervical vertebrae (C1 through C7), which are in the neck.

- There are 12 thoracic vertebrae (T1 through T12), which are located in the upper back.

- There are five lumbar vertebrae (L1 through L5), which are found in the lower back.

About This Chapter: This chapter includes text excerpted from "Spinal Cord Injury (SCI): Condition Information," *Eunice Kennedy Shriver* National Institute of Child Health and Human Development (NICHD), December 1, 2016.

- Below those are five sacral vertebrae, which are fused to form the sacrum. Finally, there are the four vertebrae of the coccyx, or tailbone.

There are two broad types of SCI, each comprising a number of different levels:

- **Tetraplegia** (formerly called "quadriplegia") generally describes the condition of a person with an SCI that is at a level anywhere from the C1 vertebra down to the T1. These individuals can experience a loss of sensation, function, or movement in their head, neck, shoulders, arms, hands, upper chest, pelvic organs, and legs.

- **Paraplegia** is the general term describing the condition of people who have lost feeling in or are not able to move the lower parts of their body. The body parts that may be affected are the chest, stomach, hips, legs, and feet. The state of an individual with an SCI level from the T2 vertebra to the S5 is usually called "paraplegic."

In addition, there are two degrees of SCI severity:

- **Complete injury** is the situation when the injury is so severe that almost all feeling (sensory function) and all ability to control movement (motor function) are lost below the area of the SCI.

- **Incomplete injury** occurs when there is some sensory or motor function below the damaged area on the spine. There are many degrees of incomplete injury.

The closer the spinal injury is to the skull, the more extensive the curtailment of the body's ability to move and feel. If the lesion is low on the spine, say, in the sacral area, it is likely that there will be a lack of feeling and movement in the thighs and lower parts of the legs, the feet, most of the external genital organs, and the anal area. But the person will be able to breathe freely and move her or his head, neck, arms, and hands. By contrast, someone with a broken neck may be almost completely incapacitated, even to the extent of requiring breathing assistance.

What Are the Symptoms of Spinal Cord Injury?

According to the American Association of Neurological Surgeons (AANS), there are many different symptoms or signs of spinal cord injury (SCI). Some of the more common signs of SCI include:

- Extreme pain or pressure in the neck, head, or back

- Tingling or loss of sensation in the hand, fingers, feet, or toes

- Partial or complete loss of control over any part of the body

- Urinary or bowel urgency, incontinence, or retention

- Difficulty with balance and walking

- Abnormal band-like sensations in the thorax—pain and pressure

- Impaired breathing after injury

- Unusual lumps on the head or spine

How Many People Are Affected by Spinal Cord Injury?

According to the National SCI Statistical Center, there are about 12,000 new cases of SCIs in the United States annually, which amounts to about 40 cases per million people. The last studies of the incidence of SCI were conducted in the 1990s, however, and so it is not known whether incidence has changed in recent years. In 2010, about a quarter of a million people in the United States were living with an SCI.

The majority of SCIs occur in young to middle-aged adults. From 1973 to 1979, the average age at injury was 28.7 years, and most injuries occurred between the ages of 16 and 30. However, demographic changes since the mid-1970s have resulted in an increase of 9 years in the median age of the U.S. population. Similarly, the average age for an SCI has increased over time. From 2005 to 2010, the average age was 40.7.

Who Is at Risk for Spinal Cord Injury?

Spinal cord injuries are typically the result of accidents and, therefore, can happen to anyone.

Factors that increase the risk of SCI include:

- Driving or riding in a car. Using a seatbelt can reduce the possibility of an SCI by 60 percent; using a seatbelt and having a functioning airbag can cut the odds of this injury by 80 percent.
- Being male. Eighty percent of SCI patients are male.
- Operating machinery without using safety equipment
- Improper or unsafe use of a ladder, which can result in a fall from the ladder
- Using drugs or alcohol while driving, operating machinery, or playing sports
- Having arthritis, osteoporosis, or other bone or joint disorders

What Causes Spinal Cord Injury, and How Does It Affect Your Body?

Spinal cord injuries result from damage to the vertebrae, ligaments, or disks of the spinal column or to the spinal cord itself.

A traumatic SCI may stem from a sudden blow to the spine that fractures, dislocates, crushes, or compresses 1 or more vertebrae. Car crashes are the leading cause of SCI among people younger than 65 years of age. Falls cause most SCIs in persons 65 years of age and older.

Since 2005, SCI has been caused by:

- Car crashes (40.4%)

- Falls (27.9%)

- Violence, including gunshot wounds (15%)

- Sport-related accidents (8%)

- Other/unknown (8.5%)

What Happens in Your Body When Your Spinal Cord Is Injured?

When an SCI occurs, the spinal cord starts to swell at the damaged area, cutting off the vital blood supply to the nerve tissue and starving it of oxygen. This sets off a cascade of devastation that affects the entire body, causing the injured spinal tissue to die, be stripped of its insulation, and be further damaged by a massive response of the immune system.

- **Blood flow.** The sluggish blood flow at the injury site begins to reduce the flow of blood in adjacent areas, which soon affects all areas of the body. The body begins to lose the ability to self-regulate, leading to drastic drops in blood pressure and heart rate.

- **Flood of neurotransmitters.** The SCI leads to an excessive release of neurotransmitters or biochemicals that let nerve cells communicate with each other. These chemicals, especially glutamate, overexcite nerve cells, killing them through a process known as "excitotoxicity." The process also kills the vital oligodendrocytes that surround and protect the spinal axons with the myelin insulation that allows the spinal nerves to transmit information to and from the brain.

- **Invasion of immune cells.** An army of cells of the immune system speeds to the damaged area of the spine. While they help by preventing infection and cleaning up dead cellular debris, they also promote inflammation. These immune cells stimulate the release of certain cytokines that, in high concentrations, can be toxic to nerve cells, especially those needed to maintain the myelin sheath around axons.

- **Onslaught of free radicals.** The inflammation caused by cells in the immune system unleashes waves of free radicals, which are highly reactive forms of oxygen molecules. These free radicals react destructively with many types of cellular molecules and, in the process, severely damage healthy nerve cells.

- **Nerve cell self-destruction.** A normally natural process of programmed cell death, known as "apoptosis," goes out of control at the injury site. The reasons are not known. Days or weeks after the injury, oligodendrocytes die from no apparent cause, reducing the integrity of the spinal cord.

Additional damage usually occurs over the days or weeks following the initial injury because of bleeding, swelling, inflammation, and accumulation of fluid in and around the spinal cord.

How Is Spinal Cord Injury Diagnosed?

Spinal cord injuries are not always immediately recognizable. The following injuries should be assessed for possible damage to the spinal cord:

- Head injuries, particularly those with trauma to the face

- Pelvic fractures

- Penetrating injuries in the area of the spine

- Injuries from falling from heights

If any of these injuries occur together with any of the symptoms mentioned above (acute head, neck, or back pain; decline of feeling in the extremities; loss of control over part of the body; urinary or bowel problems; walking difficulty; pain or pressure bands in the chest area; difficulty breathing; and head or spine lumps), then an SCI may be implicated.

A person suspected of having an SCI must be carefully transported—to prevent further injury the spine should be kept immobile—to an emergency room or trauma center. A doctor will question the person to determine the nature of the accident, and the medical staff may test the patient for sensory function and movement. If the injured person complains of neck pain, is not fully awake, or has obvious signs of weakness or neurological injury, diagnostic tests will be performed.

These tests may include:

- **Computed tomography (CT or CAT) scan.** This approach uses computers to form a series of cross-sectional images that may show the location and extent of the damage and reveal problems, such as blood clots (hematomas).

- **Magnetic resonance imaging (MRI) scan.** An MRI machine "takes a picture" of the injured area using a strong magnetic field and radio waves. A computer creates an image of the spine to reveal herniated disks and other abnormalities.

- **Myelogram.** This is an x-ray of the spine taken after a dye is injected.

- **Somatosensory evoked potential (SSEP) testing or magnetic stimulation.** Performing these tests may show if nerve signals can pass through the spinal cord.

- **Spine x-rays.** These may show fracture or damage to the bones of the spine.

On about the third day after the injury, doctors give patients a complete neurological examination to diagnose the severity of the injury and predict the likely extent of recovery. This involves testing the patient's muscle strength and ability to sense light touch and a pinprick. Doctors use the standard American Spinal Injury Association (ASIA) Impairment Scale for this diagnosis. X-rays, MRIs, or more advanced imaging techniques are also used to visualize the entire length of the spine.

The ASIA Impairment Scale has five classification levels, ranging from complete loss of neural function in the affected area to completely normal.

- A: The impairment is complete. There is no motor or sensory function left below the level of injury.

- B: The impairment is incomplete. Sensory function, but not motor function, is preserved below the neurologic level (the first normal level above the level of injury), and some sensation is preserved in the sacral segments S4 and S5.

- C: The impairment is incomplete. Motor function is preserved below the neurologic level, but more than half of the key muscles below the neurologic level have a muscle grade less than 3 (i.e., they are not strong enough to move against gravity).

- D: The impairment is incomplete. Motor function is preserved below the neurologic level, and at least half of the key muscles below the neurologic level have a muscle grade of 3 or more (i.e., the joints can be moved against gravity).

- E: The patient's functions are normal. All motor and sensory functions are unhindered.

To illustrate, a person classified as C-level on the ASIA scale functions better than a person at the B level. Not long ago, a patient might have been labeled a C4 quadriplegic. Nowadays, however, using the ASIA scale, the classification might be C4 ASIA A tetraplegic. Regarding muscle-strength grades, zero is the lowest, corresponding to complete absence of muscle movement. Five is the highest, representing full, normal strength.

What Are the Treatments for Spinal Cord Injury?

Unfortunately, at present, there are no known ways to reverse damage to the spinal cord. However, researchers are continually working on new treatments, including prostheses and medications, which may promote regeneration of nerve cells or improve the function of the nerves that remain after a spinal cord injury.

Spinal cord injury treatment currently focuses on preventing further injury and empowering people with an SCI to return to an active and productive life.

At the Scene of the Incident

Quick medical attention is critical to minimizing the effects of head, neck, or back trauma. Therefore, treatment for an SCI often begins at the scene of the injury.

Emergency personnel typically:

- Immobilize the spine as gently and quickly as possible using a rigid neck collar and a rigid carrying board
- Use the carrying board to transport the patient to the hospital

In the Emergency Room

Once the patient is at the hospital, healthcare providers focus on:

- Maintaining the person's ability to breathe
- Immobilizing the neck to prevent further spinal cord damage

Healthcare providers also may treat an acute injury with:

- **Surgery.** Doctors may use surgery to remove fluid or tissue that presses on the spinal cord (decompression laminectomy); remove bone fragments, disk fragments, or foreign objects; fuse broken spinal bones; or place spinal braces.

- **Traction.** This technique stabilizes the spine and brings it into proper alignment.

- **Methylprednisolone (Medrol).** If this steroid medication is administered within eight hours of injury, some patients experience improvement. It appears to work by reducing damage to nerve cells and decreasing inflammation near the site of injury.

- **Experimental treatments.** Scientists are pursuing research on how to halt cell death, control inflammation, and promote the repair or regeneration of nerves.

People with an SCI may benefit from rehabilitation, including:

- Physical therapy geared toward muscle strengthening, communication, and mobility

- Use of assistive devices, such as wheelchairs, walkers, and leg braces

- Use of adaptive devices for communication

- Occupational therapy focused on fine motor skills

- Techniques for self-grooming and bladder and bowel management

- Coping strategies for dealing with spasticity and pain

- Vocational therapy to help people get back to work with the use of assistive devices, if needed

- Recreational therapy, such as sports and social activities

- Improved strategies for exercise and healthy diets (obesity and diabetes are potential risk factors for persons with SCI)

- Functional electrical stimulation for assistance with restoration of neuromuscular function, sensory function, or autonomic function (e.g., bladder, bowel, or respiratory function).

What Conditions Are Associated with Spinal Cord Injury?

Spinal cord injury is associated with many secondary conditions that have significant impacts on medical rehabilitation management, long-term outcome, and quality of life.

Secondary conditions associated with SCIs include:

- Breathing problems

- Bowel and bladder problems, including overactive bladder and incontinence

- Heart problems

- Pressure sores

- Sexual function problems

- Pain

- Blood clots

- Impaired muscle coordination (or spasticity)

- Pneumonia

- Hyperreflexia, which causes a potentially lethal increase in blood pressure

- Increased likelihood of certain cancers, including bladder cancer

Adjusting

Adjustment is a big part of dealing with a spinal cord injury. Adjustment means getting used to something new and also making changes to better handle something new. Each person who is injured adjusts in her or his own way. For teens, coping with changes after an injury can be even harder. This is because, as a teen, you also are coping with the change from childhood to adulthood.

Adjusting to your injury likely will be easier if you:

- Set some personal goals, such as working hard in each therapy session to gain strength or getting back into a club at school

- Make an effort to stay in touch with your old friends and try making new friends at your physical therapy sessions

- Try your hardest to talk through any problems that come up between you and your family members since your relationships may change during this time

(Source: "Spinal Cord Injury," girlshealth.gov, Office on Women's Health (OWH).)

Chapter 15

Concussions

What Is Concussion?

A concussion is a type of brain injury. It involves a short loss of normal brain function. It happens when a blow to the head or body causes your head and brain to move rapidly back and forth. This sudden movement can cause the brain to bounce around or twist in the skull, creating chemical changes in your brain. It can also stretch and damage your brain cells.

Sometimes, people call a concussion a "mild" brain injury. It is important to understand that while concussions may not be life-threatening, they can still be serious.

What Causes Concussion

Concussions are a common type of sports injury. Other causes of concussions include blows to the head, bumping your head when you fall, being violently shaken, and car accidents.

What Are the Symptoms of Concussion?

Symptoms of a concussion may not start right away; they may start days or weeks after the injury. Symptoms may include a headache or neck pain. You may also have nausea, ringing in your ears, dizziness, or tiredness. You may feel dazed or not your normal self for several days or weeks after the injury. Consult your healthcare professional if any of your symptoms get worse or if you have more serious symptoms, such as:

- Convulsions or seizures

- Drowsiness or an inability to wake up

About This Chapter: This chapter includes text excerpted from "Concussion," MedlinePlus, National Institutes of Health (NIH), June 28, 2018.

- A headache that gets worse and does not go away

- Weakness, numbness, or decreased coordination

- Repeated vomiting or nausea

- Confusion

- Slurred speech

- Loss of consciousness

Immediately after a concussion, the brain is especially vulnerable to having a second, more serious injury. But, it is not clear why—or how long that vulnerable period lasts. Studies have found that the risk for a second injury is greatest in the 10 days following an initial concussion. If you suspect that someone has a concussion, make sure they stop whatever activity they are doing, especially if they are involved in a sport. Their brain dysfunction might not only cloud their thinking, but can also slow reaction times and affect their balance so they become more likely to have another injury.

(Source: "Bang to the Brain: What We Know about Concussions," NIH News in Health, *National Institutes of Health (NIH).)*

How Is Concussion Diagnosed?

To diagnose a concussion, your healthcare provider will do a physical exam and will ask about your injury. You will most likely have a neurological exam, which checks your vision, balance, coordination, and reflexes. Your healthcare provider may also evaluate your memory and thinking. In some cases, you may also have a scan of the brain, such as a computed tomography (CT) scan or a magnetic resonance imaging (MRI). A scan can check for bleeding or inflammation in the brain, as well as skull fractures.

What Is the Prognosis for Concussion?

Most people recover fully after a concussion, but it can take some time. Rest is very important after a concussion because it helps the brain to heal. In the very beginning, you may need to limit physical activities or activities that involve a lot of concentration, such as studying, working on the computer, or playing video games. Doing these may cause concussion symptoms (such as headache or tiredness) to come back or get worse. Then when your healthcare provider says that it is okay, you can start to return to your normal activities slowly.

Chapter 16

Traumatic Brain Injury

Traumatic brain injury (TBI) is a serious public-health problem in the United States. Each year, TBIs contribute to a substantial number of deaths and cases of permanent disability. In 2014, there were approximately 2.87 million TBI-related emergency department visits, hospitalizations, and deaths in the United States, including over 837,000 of these health events among children.

Get the Facts

Traumatic brain injury is a major cause of death and disability in the United States. From 2006 to 2014, the number of TBI-related emergency department visits, hospitalizations, and deaths increased by 53 percent. In 2014, an average of 155 people in the United States died each day from injuries that include a TBI. Those who survive a TBI can face effects that last a few days or the rest of their lives. Effects of TBI can include impairments related to thinking or memory, movement, sensation (e.g., vision or hearing), or emotional functioning (e.g., personality changes, depression). These issues not only affect individuals but also can have lasting effects on families and communities.

What Is a Traumatic Brain Injury?

A TBI is caused by a bump, blow, or jolt to the head that disrupts the normal function of the brain. Not all blows or jolts to the head result in a TBI. The severity of a TBI may range from "mild" (i.e., a brief change in mental status or consciousness) to "severe" (i.e., an extended

About This Chapter: This chapter includes text excerpted from "Basic Information about Traumatic Brain Injury," Centers for Disease Control and Prevention (CDC), March 6, 2019.

period of unconsciousness or memory loss after the injury). Most TBIs that occur each year are mild, commonly called "concussions."

How Big Is the Problem of Traumatic Brain Injury?

- In 2014, about 2.87 million TBI-related emergency department (ED) visits, hospitalizations, and deaths occurred in the United States, including over 837,000 of these health events among children.

- TBI contributed to the deaths of 56,800 people, including 2,529 deaths among children.

- TBI was diagnosed in approximately 288,000 hospitalizations, including over 23,000 among children. These consisted of TBI alone or TBI in combination with other injuries.

- In 2014, an estimated 812,000 children (17 years of age or younger) were treated in the United States. EDs for concussion or TBI, alone or in combination with other injuries.

- Over the span of 8 years (2006 to 2014), while age-adjusted rates of TBI-related ED visits increased by 54 percent, hospitalization rates decreased by 8 percent and death rates decreased by 6 percent.

What Are the Leading Causes of Traumatic Brain Injury?

- In 2014, falls were the leading cause of TBI. Falls accounted for almost half (48%) of all TBI-related emergency department visits. Falls disproportionately affect children and older adults:

- Almost half (49%) of TBI-related ED visits among children between the ages of 0 and 17 were caused by falls.

- 4 in 5 (81%) TBI-related ED visits in adults 65 years of age and older were caused by falls.

- Being struck by or against an object was the second leading cause of TBI-related ED visits, accounting for about 17 percent of all TBI-related ED visits in the United States in 2014.

- Over 1 in 4 (28%) TBI-related ED visits in children 17 years of age or younger were caused by being struck by or against an object.

- Falls and motor vehicle crashes were the first and second leading causes of all TBI-related hospitalizations (52% and 20%, respectively).

- Intentional self-harm was the first leading cause of TBI-related deaths (33%) in 2014.

Risk Factors of Traumatic Brain Injury

Among TBI-related deaths in 2014:

- Rates were highest for persons 75 years of age and older.

- The leading cause of TBI-related death varied by age:

  - Falls were the leading cause of death for persons 65 years of age or older.

  - Intentional self-harm was the leading cause of death for persons 45 to 64 years of age.

  - Motor vehicle crashes were the leading cause of death for persons 15 to 24 years of age, 25 to 34 years of age, and adults 75 years of age or older.

  - Homicide was the leading cause of death for children between the ages of 0 and 4 years.

Among TBI-related ED visits and hospitalizations in 2014:

- Hospitalization rates were highest among persons 75 years of age and older.

- Rates of ED visits were highest for persons 75 years of age and older and children between 0 and 4 years of age.

- The leading cause of TBI-related ED visits varied by age:

  - Falls were the leading cause of ED visits among young children between 0 and 4 years of age and among adults 65 years of age and older.

  - Being struck by or against an object was highest among those between 5 and 14 years of age.

- The leading cause of TBI-related hospitalizations varied by age:

  - Falls were the leading cause of hospitalizations among children 0 to 17 years of age and adults 55 years of age and older.

  - Motor vehicle crashes were the leading cause of hospitalizations for adolescents and adults between 15 and 44 years of age.

Symptoms of Traumatic Brain Injury
What Are the Symptoms of Traumatic Brain Injury?

Most people with a TBI recover well from symptoms experienced at the time of the injury. Most TBIs that occur each year are mild, commonly called "concussions," which is a mild TBI. But for some people, symptoms can last for days, weeks, or longer. In general, recovery may be slower among older adults, young children, and teens. Those who have had a TBI in the past are also at risk of having another one. Some people may also find that it takes longer to recover if they have another TBI.

Table 16.1. Categories of Traumatic Brain Injury

Thinking/ Remembering	Physical	Emotional/Mood	Sleep
Difficulty thinking clearly	Headache, fuzzy or blurry vision	Irritability	Sleeping more than usual
Feeling slowed down	Nausea or vomiting (early on), dizziness	Sadness	Sleep less than usual
Difficulty concentrating	Sensitivity to noise or light, balance problems	More emotional	Trouble falling asleep
Difficulty remembering new information	Feeling tired, having no energy	Nervousness or anxiety	

Some of these symptoms may appear right away. Others may not be noticed for days or months after the injury, or until the person resumes their everyday life. Sometimes, people do not recognize or admit that they are having problems. Others may not understand their problems and how the symptoms they are experiencing impact their daily activities.

The signs and symptoms of a concussion can be difficult to sort out. Early on, problems may be overlooked by the person with the concussion, family members, or doctors. People may look fine even though they are acting or feeling differently.

When to Seek Immediate Medical Attention
Danger Signs in Adults

In rare cases, a dangerous blood clot that crowds the brain against the skull can develop. The people checking on you should take you to an emergency department right away if you:

- Have a headache that gets worse and does not go away

- Experience weakness, numbness, or decreased coordination

- Have repeated vomiting or nausea

- Slur your speech

- Look very drowsy or cannot wake up

- Have one pupil (the black part in the middle of the eye) larger than the other

- Have convulsions or seizures

- Cannot recognize people or places

- Are getting more and more confused, restless, or agitated

- Have unusual behavior

- Lose consciousness

Danger Signs in Children

A child or teen should be taken to the emergency department right away if they received a bump, blow, or jolt to the head or body, and:

- Have any of the danger signs for adults listed above

- Will not stop crying and are inconsolable

- Will not nurse or eat

Response to Concussion
What Should I Do If a Concussion Occurs?

People with a concussion need to be seen by a healthcare professional. If you think you or someone you know has a concussion, contact your healthcare professional. Your healthcare professional can evaluate your concussion and determine if you need to be referred to a neurologist, neuropsychologist, neurosurgeon, or specialist in rehabilitation (such as a speech pathologist) for specialized care. Getting help soon after the injury by trained specialists may improve recovery.

What to Expect When You See a Healthcare Professional

While most people are seen in an emergency department or medical office, some people must stay in the hospital overnight. Your healthcare professional may do a scan of your brain (such as a computed tomography (CT) scan) or other tests. Additional tests might be necessary, such as tests of your learning, memory, concentration, and problem solving. These tests are called "neuropsychological tests" or "neurocognitive tests," and they can help your healthcare professional identify the effects of a concussion. Even if the concussion does not show up on these tests, you may still have a concussion.

Your healthcare professional will send you home with important instructions to follow. Be sure to follow all of your healthcare professional's instructions carefully.

If you are taking medications—prescription, over-the-counter (OTC) medicines, or "natural remedies"—or if you drink alcohol or take illicit drugs, tell your healthcare professional. Also, tell your healthcare professional if you are taking blood thinners (anticoagulant drugs), such as Coumadin and aspirin, because they can increase the chance of complications.

Recovery from Concussion

Most children with a concussion feel better within a couple of weeks. However, for some, symptoms will last for a month or longer. Concussion symptoms may appear during the normal healing process or as their regular activities resume. If there are any symptoms that concern you or are getting worse, be sure to seek medical care as soon as possible.

What Steps Should You Take to Feel Better?

Making short-term changes to your daily activities can help you to get back to a regular routine more quickly. As you begin to feel better, you can slowly remove these changes. Use your symptoms to guide your return to normal activities. If your symptoms do not worsen during an activity, then this activity is okay for you. If symptoms worsen, then you should cut back on how much you can do that activity without experiencing symptoms. It is important to remember that each concussion and each person is unique, so recovery should be customized based on a person's symptoms.

Rest

A person recovering from a concussion should take it easy the first few days after the injury when symptoms are more severe.

- Early on, limit physical and thinking/remembering activities to avoid symptoms getting worse.

- Avoid activities that put a person at risk for another injury to the head and brain.

- Get a good night's sleep, and take naps during the day as needed.

Light Activity

As a person starts to feel better, she or he can gradually return to regular (nonstrenuous) activities.

- Find relaxing activities at home.

- Return to school gradually.

- Get maximum nighttime sleep. Avoid screen time and loud music before bed, sleep in a dark room, and keep to a fixed bedtime and wake up schedule.

- Reduce daytime naps or return to a regular daytime nap schedule (as appropriate for their age).

Moderate Activity

When symptoms are mild and nearly gone, an individual can return to most regular activities.

- Help a person take breaks only if concussion symptoms worsen.

- Return to a regular school schedule.

Back to Regular Activity

Recovery from a concussion is when a child or teen is able to do all of their regular activities without experiencing any symptoms.

Also, be sure to:

- Keep all follow-up appointments.

- Ask the doctor or nurse about safe over-the-counter (OTC) or prescription medications to help with symptoms (e.g., Ibuprofen or acetaminophen for headache).

- Limit the number of soft drinks or caffeinated items to help bring about rest.

Postconcussive Syndrome

While most children and teens with a concussion feel better within a couple of weeks, some will have symptoms for months or longer. Talk with the healthcare provider if the concussion symptoms do not go away or if they get worse after returning to the regular activities.

If concussion symptoms last for weeks to months after the injury, the medical provider may talk about postconcussive syndrome (PCS). While rare after only one concussion, PCS is believed to occur most commonly in patients with a history of multiple concussions.

There are many people who can help in recovery. If things do not get better, tell your medical provider.

What Are the Potential Effects of Traumatic Brain Injury?

The severity of a traumatic brain injury may range from "mild" (i.e., a brief change in mental status or consciousness) to "severe" (i.e., an extended period of unconsciousness or amnesia after the injury).

A TBI can cause a wide range of functional short- or long-term changes affecting:

- **Thinking** (i.e., memory and reasoning)

- **Sensation** (i.e., sight and balance)

- **Language** (i.e., communication, expression, and understanding)

- **Emotion** (i.e., depression, anxiety, personality changes, aggression, acting out, and social inappropriateness)

A TBI can also cause epilepsy and increase the risk for conditions, such as Alzheimer disease (AD), Parkinson disease (PD), and other brain disorders.

Tips to Help Aid in Recovery

- Get a lot of rest. Do not rush back to daily activities, such as work or school.
- Avoid doing anything that could cause another blow or jolt to the head.
- Ask your healthcare professional when it is safe to drive a car, ride a bike, or use heavy equipment. Your ability to react may be slower after a brain injury.
- Only take medications your healthcare provider has approved. Do not drink alcohol until your healthcare provider says it is okay.
- Write things down if you have a hard time remembering.
- You may need help to relearn skills you lost. Your healthcare professional can help arrange for these services.

About 75 percent of TBIs that occur each year are concussions or other forms of mild TBI.

Repeated mild TBIs occurring over an extended period of time can result in cumulative neurological and cognitive deficits. Repeated mild TBIs occurring within a short period of time (i.e., hours, days, or weeks) can be catastrophic or fatal.

Prevention of Traumatic Brain Injury

There are many ways to reduce the chances of sustaining a traumatic brain injury.

You Can Prevent Traumatic Brain Injury

- Buckle up. Wear a seat belt every time you drive—or ride—in a motor vehicle.

- Never drive while under the influence of alcohol or drugs.

- Wear a helmet, or appropriate headgear, when you:

  - Ride a bike, motorcycle, snowmobile, scooter, or use an all-terrain vehicle

  - Play a contact sport, such as football, ice hockey, or boxing

  - Use in-line skates or ride a skateboard

  - Bat and run bases in baseball or softball

  - Ride a horse

  - Ski or snowboard

- Prevent older adult falls.

  - Talk to your doctor to evaluate your risk for falling, and ask about specific things you can do to reduce your risk for a fall.

  - Ask your doctor or pharmacist to review your medicines to see if any might make you dizzy or sleepy. This should include prescription medicines, OTC medicines, herbal supplements, and vitamins.

  - Have your eyes checked at least once a year, and be sure to update your eyeglasses if needed.

  - Do strength and balance exercises to make your legs stronger and improve your balance.

  - Make your home safer.

- Make living and play areas safer for children
  - Install window guards to keep young children from falling out of open windows.
  - Use safety gates at the top and bottom of stairs when young children are around.
  - Make sure a child's playground has soft material under it, such as hardwood mulch or sand.

Severe Traumatic Brain Injury

Each year, TBI causes a substantial number of deaths and leads to lifelong disability for many Americans. In fact, TBIs contribute to about 30 percent of all injury deaths in the United States. In 2014, there were:

- Approximately 2.5 million TBI-related emergency department visits
- Approximately 288,000 hospitalizations
- Nearly 57,000 deaths related to TBI

The effects of a TBI can vary significantly, depending on the severity. Individuals with a mild TBI generally experience short-term symptoms and feel better within a couple of weeks, whereas individuals with a moderate or severe TBI may have long-term or lifelong effects from the injury.

A severe TBI not only impacts the life of an individual and their family, but it also has a large societal and economic toll. The lifetime economic cost of TBI, including direct and indirect medical costs, was estimated to be approximately $76.5 billion (in 2010 dollars). Additionally, the cost of fatal TBIs and TBIs requiring hospitalization, many of which are severe, account for approximately 90 percent of total TBI medical costs. Falls are one of the leading causes of TBI-related ED visits, hospitalizations, and deaths, and data shows that over half of fall-related TBIs were among the youngest (between 0 and 4 years of age) and oldest age groups (75 years of age and older).

Potential Effects of Severe Traumatic Brain Injury

The long-term effects of a TBI have been described as being similar to the effects of a chronic disease. Individuals who experience mild TBI are more likely to recover from their initial injury symptoms, although some individuals experience longer-term effects. Individuals who experience more severe TBIs are more likely to have lasting effects from the injury.

A TBI may lead to a wide range of short- or long-term issues affecting:

- **Cognitive function** (attention and memory)

- **Motor function** (extremity weakness, impaired coordination and balance)

- **Sensation** (hearing, vision, impaired perception and touch)

- **Behavior** (emotional regulation, depression, anxiety, aggression, impairments in behavioral control, personality changes)

A severe TBI may lead to death or result in an extended period of unconsciousness (coma) or amnesia. Individuals may experience significant changes in thinking and behavior. Moderate-to-severe TBI may also result in a reduced lifespan.

The consequences of severe TBI can affect all aspects of an individual's life, including relationships with family and friends, the ability to progress at school or work, doing household tasks, driving, or participating in other daily activities.

Chapter 17

Choking

Food or small objects can cause choking if they get caught in your throat and block your airway. This keeps oxygen from getting to your lungs and brain. If your brain goes without oxygen for more than four minutes, you could have brain damage or die.

Young children are at an especially high risk of choking. They can choke on foods, such as hot dogs, nuts, and grapes, and on small objects, such as toy pieces and coins.

When someone is choking, quick action can be lifesaving.

You can prevent yourself from choking by:

- Sitting up while eating (no lying down)
- Sitting in a high chair or a safe place
- Avoiding eating in the car

(Source: "Choking Hazards," Centers for Disease Control and Prevention (CDC).)

About This Chapter: Text in this chapter begins with excerpts from "Choking," MedlinePlus, National Institutes of Health (NIH), March 31, 2016; Text under the heading "What Is Cardiopulmonary Resuscitation and When Should You Use It?" is excerpted from "Three Things You May Not Know about Cardiopulmonary Resuscitation," Centers for Disease Control and Prevention (CDC), October 9, 2018; Text under the heading "Abdominal Thrusts" is excerpted from "5 Practical Skills for the Holiday 'Host(ess)' with the Mostest," Centers for Disease Control and Prevention (CDC), April 15, 2019.

What Is Cardiopulmonary Resuscitation and When Should You Use It?

Cardiopulmonary resuscitation (CPR) is an emergency procedure that can help save a person's life if their breathing or heart stops. When a person's heart stops beating, they are in cardiac arrest. During cardiac arrest, the heart cannot pump blood to the rest of the body, including to the brain and lungs. Death can happen in minutes without treatment. CPR uses chest compressions to mimic how the heart pumps. These compressions help keep blood flowing throughout the body.

Cardiac arrest is not the same as a heart attack. A heart attack happens when blood flow to the heart is blocked. A person having a heart attack is still talking and breathing. This person does not need CPR, but they do need to get to the hospital right away. Heart attack increases the risk of going into cardiac arrest.

Cardiopulmonary Resuscitation Saves Lives

About 9 in 10 people who have cardiac arrest outside the hospital die. But, CPR can help improve those odds. If it is performed in the first few minutes of cardiac arrest, CPR can double or triple a person's chance of survival.

Certain people, including people in low-income, Black, and Hispanic neighborhoods, are less likely to receive CPR from bystanders than people in high-income, White neighborhoods. Women may also be less likely to receive CPR if they experience cardiac arrest in a public place.

How Can You Tell Whether Someone Is in Cardiac Arrest?

- The person is unresponsive, even if you shake or shout at them.
- The person is not breathing or only gasping.

If you see someone in cardiac arrest, call 911 right away and start CPR. Keep doing CPR until medical professionals arrive.

Most cardiac arrests happen outside of the hospital, either at home or in public places. If CPR is performed in the first few minutes of cardiac arrest, it can double or triple a person's chance of survival.

Cardiac Arrests Often Happen at Home

About 350,000 cardiac arrests happen outside of hospitals each year, and about 7 in 10 of those happen at home. Unfortunately, about half of the people who experience cardiac arrests at home do not get the help they need from bystanders before an ambulance arrives.

If you see cardiac arrest happen, call 911 right away and perform CPR until medical professionals arrive.

You Do Not Need Formal Training to Perform Cardiopulmonary Resuscitation

You do not need a special certification or formal training to perform CPR, but you do need education. If cardiac arrest happens to someone near you, do not be afraid—just be prepared. Follow these steps if you see someone in cardiac arrest:

- **Call 911 right away.** If another bystander is nearby, save time by asking that person to call 911 and look for an automated external defibrillator (AED) while you begin CPR. AEDs are portable machines that can electrically shock the heart and cause it to start beating again.

- **Give CPR.** Push down hard and fast in the center of the chest at a rate of 100 to 120 pushes a minute. Let the chest come back up to its normal position after each push. The American Heart Association (AHA) recommends timing your pushes to the beat of the song "Stayin' Alive." This method of CPR is called "hands-only" and does not involve breathing into the person's mouth.

- Continue giving CPR until medical professionals arrive or until a person with formal CPR training can take over.

Abdominal Thrusts

Know how to help someone who is choking. Giving abdominal thrusts, also known as "Heimlich maneuver," is a method of applying pressure to remove an obstruction, such as a piece of food, from a person's windpipe. Along with hands-only CPR, knowing how to respond in a choking emergency is a basic life-saving skill that anyone can learn and teach to others.

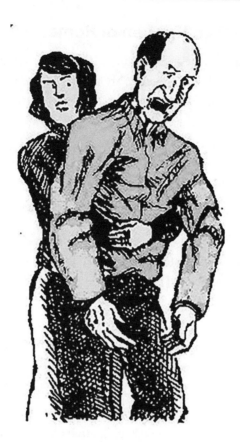

Figure 17.1. *Abdominal Thrusts (Source: "First Aid Basics," Agricultural Research Service (ARS), U.S. Department of Agriculture (USDA).)*

If you suspect a person is choking and/or see someone giving the universal sign of choking—holding their neck with one or both hands—immediately take the following steps:

- Ask the person if they are choking. DO NOT perform first aid if the person is coughing forcefully and is able to speak.

- If they are unable to speak, perform abdominal thrusts:

  - Stand behind the person and wrap your arms around the person's waist. For a child, you may have to kneel.

  - Make a fist with one hand. Place the thumb side of your fist just above the person's navel, well below the breastbone.

  - Grasp the fist tightly with your other hand.

- Make a quick, upward and inward thrust with your fist.

- Check if the object was dislodged.

- Continue thrusts until the object is dislodged or the person loses consciousness.

- Call 911 if the person loses consciousness. Always call 911 in a life-threatening emergency.

Chapter 18

Alcohol Overdose

Celebrating at parties, cheering a favorite sports team, and enjoying get-togethers after work are common ways to relax or be with friends. For some people, these occasions may also include drinking—even binge or extreme binge drinking (also known as "high-intensity drinking"). And when that happens, the results can be deadly.

Drinking too much and too quickly can lead to significant impairments in motor coordination, decision-making, impulse control, and other functions, increasing the risk of harm. Continuing to drink despite clear signs of significant impairments can result in an alcohol overdose.

What Is an Alcohol Overdose?

An alcohol overdose occurs when there is so much alcohol in the bloodstream that areas of the brain controlling basic life-support functions—such as breathing, heart rate, and temperature control—begin to shut down. Symptoms of alcohol overdose include mental confusion; difficulty remaining conscious; vomiting; seizures; trouble breathing; a slow heart rate; clammy skin; dulled responses, such as no gag reflex (which prevents choking); and an extremely low body temperature. Alcohol overdose can lead to permanent brain damage or death.

What tips the balance from drinking that produces impairment to drinking that puts one's life in jeopardy varies among individuals. Age, sensitivity to alcohol (tolerance), sex, speed of drinking, medications you are taking, and amount of food eaten can all be factors.

About This Chapter: This chapter includes text excerpted from "Understanding the Dangers of Alcohol Overdose," National Institute on Alcohol Abuse and Alcoholism (NIAAA), October 2018.

Alcohol use and taking opioids or sedative-hypnotics, such as sleep and antianxiety medications, can increase your risk of an overdose. Examples of these medications include sleep aids, such as zolpidem (Ambien) and eszopiclone (Lunesta), and benzodiazepines, such as diazepam (Valium) and alprazolam (Xanax). Even drinking alcohol while taking over-the-counter (OTC) antihistamines can be dangerous. Using alcohol with opioid pain relievers, such as oxycodone and morphine, or illicit opioids, such as heroin, is also a very dangerous combination. As with alcohol, these drugs suppress areas in the brain that control vital functions, such as breathing. Ingesting alcohol and other drugs together intensify their individual effects and could produce an overdose with even moderate amounts of alcohol.

Who May Be at Risk?

Anyone who consumes too much alcohol too quickly may be in danger of an alcohol overdose. This is especially true of individuals who engage in binge drinking, defined as a pattern of drinking that brings blood alcohol concentration (BAC) to .08 percent or higher,* typically occurring after a woman consumes four drinks or a man consumes five drinks in about two hours, as well as extreme binge drinking, which is defined as drinking two or more times the binge-drinking thresholds for women and men.

Teenagers and young adults who drink may be at particular risk for alcohol overdose. Research shows that teens and college-aged young adults often engage in binge drinking and extreme binge drinking. Drinking such large quantities of alcohol can overwhelm the body's ability to break down and clear alcohol from the bloodstream. This leads to rapid increases in BAC, and it significantly impairs brain and other bodily functions.

A BAC of .08 percent corresponds to .08 grams per deciliter, or .08 grams per 100 milliliters.

As Blood Alcohol Concentration Increases, So Do the Risks

As BAC increases, so does the effect of alcohol—as well as the risk of harm. Even small increases in BAC can decrease motor coordination, make a person feel sick, and cloud judgment. This can increase an individual's risk of being injured from falls or car crashes, experiencing acts of violence, and engaging in unprotected or unintended sex. When BAC reaches high levels, amnesia (blackouts), loss of consciousness (passing out), and death can occur.

A person's BAC can continue to rise even when she or he stops drinking or is unconscious. Alcohol in the stomach and intestine continues to enter the bloodstream and circulate throughout the body.

It is dangerous to assume that an unconscious person will be fine by sleeping it off. One potential danger of alcohol overdose is choking on one's own vomit. Alcohol at very high levels can hinder signals in the brain that control automatic responses, such as the gag reflex. With no gag reflex, a person who drinks to the point of passing out is in danger of choking on her or his vomit and dying from a lack of oxygen (i.e., asphyxiation). Even if the person survives, an alcohol overdose like this can lead to long-lasting brain damage.

Critical Signs and Symptoms of an Alcohol Overdose

- Mental confusion, stupor
- Difficulty remaining conscious or an inability to wake up
- Vomiting
- Seizures
- Slow breathing (fewer than 8 breaths per minute)
- Irregular breathing (10 seconds or more between breaths)
- A slow heart rate
- Clammy skin
- Dulled responses, such as no gag reflex
- Extremely low body temperature, a blueish skin color, or paleness

---

Know the Danger Signs and Act Quickly

Know the danger signals and if you suspect that someone has an alcohol overdose, call 911 for help immediately. Do not wait for the person to have all the symptoms, and be aware that a person who has passed out can die. Do not play doctor—cold showers, hot coffee, and walking do not reverse the effects of alcohol overdose and could actually make things worse.

While waiting for medical help to arrive:

- Be prepared to provide information to the responders, including the type and amount of alcohol the person drank; other drugs she or he took if known; and any health information that you know about the person, such as medications that they are currently taking, allergies to medications, and any existing health conditions.

- Do not leave an intoxicated person alone, as she or he is at risk of getting injured from falling or choking. Keep the person on the ground in a sitting or partially upright position rather than in a chair.

- Help a person who is vomiting. Have her or him lean forward to prevent choking. If a person is unconscious or lying down, roll her or him onto one side with an ear toward the ground to prevent choking.

Stay alert to keep your friends and family safe. And remember—you can avoid the risk of an alcohol overdose by drinking responsibly if you choose to drink or by not drinking at all.

Chapter 19

Opioid Overdose

What Are Opioids?

Opioids, sometimes called "narcotics," are a type of drug. They include strong prescription pain relievers, such as oxycodone, hydrocodone, fentanyl, and tramadol. The illegal drug heroin is also an opioid.

A healthcare provider may give you a prescription opioid to reduce pain after you have had a major injury or surgery. You may get them if you have severe pain from a health condition, such as cancer. Some healthcare providers prescribe them for chronic pain.

Prescription opioids used for pain relief are generally safe when taken for a short time and as prescribed by your healthcare provider. However, people who take opioids are at risk for opioid dependence and addiction, as well as an overdose. These risks increase when opioids are misused. Misuse means that you are not taking the medicines according to your provider's instructions, you are using them to get high, or you are taking someone else's opioids.

What Is an Opioid Overdose?

Opioids affect the part of the brain that regulates breathing. When people take high doses of opioids, it can lead to an overdose, which includes the slowing or stopping of breathing and sometimes death.

About This Chapter: This chapter includes text excerpted from "Opioid Overdose," MedlinePlus, National Institutes of Health (NIH), August 27, 2018.

What Causes an Opioid Overdose

An opioid overdose can happen for a variety of reasons, including if you:

- Take an opioid to get high

- Take an extra dose of a prescription opioid or take it too often (either accidentally or on purpose)

- Mix an opioid with other medicines, illegal drugs, or alcohol. An overdose can be fatal when mixing an opioid and certain anxiety treatment medicines, such as Xanax or Valium.

- Take an opioid medicine that was prescribed for someone else. Children are especially at risk of an accidental overdose if they take medicine not intended for them.

There is also a risk of overdose if you are getting medication-assisted treatment (MAT). MAT is a treatment for opioid abuse and addiction. Many of the medicines used for MAT are controlled substances that can be misused.

Who Is at Risk for an Opioid Overdose?

Anyone who takes an opioid can be at risk of an overdose, but you are at a higher risk if you:

- Take illegal opioids

- Take more opioid medicine than you are prescribed

- Combine opioids with other medicines and/or alcohol

- Have certain medical conditions, such as sleep apnea or reduced kidney or liver function

What Are the Signs of an Opioid Overdose?

The signs of an opioid overdose include:

- The person's face is extremely pale and/or feels clammy to the touch.

- Their body goes limp.

- Their fingernails or lips have a purple or blue color.

- They start vomiting or making gurgling noises.

- They cannot be awakened or are unable to speak.

- Their breathing or heartbeat slows or stops.

What Should I Do If I Think That Someone Is Having an Opioid Overdose?

If you think someone is having an opioid overdose:

- Call 911 immediately.

- Administer naloxone, if it is available. Naloxone is a safe medication that can quickly stop an opioid overdose. It can be injected into the muscle or sprayed into the nose to rapidly block the effects of the opioid on the body.

- Try to keep the person awake and breathing.

- Lay the person on their side to prevent choking.

- Stay with the person until emergency workers arrive.

Can an Opioid Overdose Be Prevented?

There are steps you can take to help prevent an overdose:

- Take your medicine exactly as prescribed by your healthcare provider. Do not take more medicine at once or take medicine more often than you are supposed to.

- Never mix pain medicines with alcohol, sleeping pills, or illegal substances.

- Store medicine safely where children or pets cannot reach it. Consider using a medicine lock box. Besides keeping children safe, it also prevents someone who lives with you or visits your house from stealing your medicines.

- Dispose of unused medicine promptly.

Naloxone

Naloxone is a medication designed to rapidly reverse opioid overdose. It is an opioid antagonist—meaning that it binds to opioid receptors and can reverse and block the effects of other opioids. It can very quickly restore normal respiration to a person whose breathing has slowed or stopped as a result of overdosing with heroin or prescription opioid pain medications.

(Source: "Opioid Overdose Reversal with Naloxone (Narcan, Evzio)," National Institute on Drug Abuse (NIDA).)

- If you take an opioid, it is also important to teach your family and friends how to respond to an overdose. If you are at a high risk for an overdose, ask your healthcare provider about whether you need a prescription for naloxone.

Part Three
Motor Vehicle Safety

Chapter 20

Teen Drivers: The Facts

Motor vehicle crashes are the leading cause of death for U.S. teens. Fortunately, teen motor vehicle crashes are preventable, and proven strategies can improve the safety of young drivers on the road.

How Big Is the Teen Motor Vehicle Crashes Problem?

In 2016, 2,433 teens in the United States between 16 and 19 years of age were killed, and 292,742 were treated in emergency departments for injuries suffered in motor vehicle crashes. That means that 6 teens between 16 and 19 years of age died every day due to motor vehicle crashes, and hundreds more were injured.

In 2016, young people between 16 and 19 years of age represented 6.5 percent of the U.S. population. However, they accounted for an estimated $13.6 billion (8.4%) of the total costs of motor vehicle injuries.

Who Is Most at Risk for Teen Motor Vehicle Crashes?

The risk of motor vehicle crashes is higher among 16- to 19-year-olds than among any other age group. In fact, per mile driven, teen drivers between 16 and 19 years of age are nearly 3 times more likely than drivers 20 years of age and older to be in a fatal crash.

About This Chapter: This chapter includes text excerpted from "Teen Drivers: Get the Facts," Centers for Disease Control and Prevention (CDC), October 19, 2018.

Among teen drivers, those at an especially high risk for motor vehicle crashes are:

- **Males.** In 2016, the motor vehicle death rate for male drivers between 16 and 19 years of age was 2 times that of their female counterparts.

- **Teens driving with teen passengers.** The presence of teen passengers increases the crash risk of unsupervised teen drivers. This risk increases with the number of teen passengers.

- **Newly licensed teens.** Crash risk is particularly high during the first months of licensure. The fatal crash rate per mile driven is nearly twice as high for 16- to 17-year-olds when compared with 18- to 19-year-olds.

What Factors Put Teen Drivers at Risk

Teens are more likely than older drivers to underestimate dangerous situations or not be able to recognize hazardous situations. Teens are also more likely than adults to make critical decision errors that lead to serious crashes.

Teens are more likely than older drivers to speed and allow shorter headways (the distance from the front of one vehicle to the front of the next). In 2016, 49 percent of teen deaths from motor vehicle crashes occurred between 3 p.m. and midnight, and 53 percent occurred on Friday, Saturday, or Sunday.

Compared with other age groups, teens have among the lowest rates of seat belt use. In 2017, only 59 percent of high-school students reported that they always wear seat belts when riding as passengers.

At all levels of blood alcohol concentration (BAC), the risk of involvement in a motor vehicle crash is greater for teens than for older drivers.

Among male drivers between 15 and 20 years of age who were involved in fatal crashes in 2016, 32 percent were speeding at the time of the crash, and 21 percent had been drinking. In 2016, 15 percent of drivers between 16 and 20 years of age involved in fatal motor vehicle crashes had a BAC of .08 percent or higher.

In the 2017 National Youth Risk Behavior Survey (YRBS), 16.5 percent of high school students reported that, within the previous month, they had ridden with a driver who had been drinking alcohol. Among students who drove, 5.5 percent reported having driven after drinking alcohol within the same 1-month period.

In 2016, 58 percent of drivers between 15 and 20 years of age who were killed in motor vehicle crashes after drinking and driving were not wearing a seatbelt.

How Can Deaths and Injuries Resulting from Crashes Involving Teen Drivers Be Prevented?

You should be aware of the leading causes of teen crashes. Most important among them being:

- Driver inexperience

- Driving with teen passengers

- Nighttime driving

- Not using seat belts

- Distracted driving

- Drowsy driving

- Reckless driving

- Impaired driving

There are proven methods to help teens become safer drivers.

Research has shown what can be done to keep teen drivers safe from each of these risks.

Seat Belts

Of the teens (between 16 and 19 years of age) who died in passenger vehicle crashes in 2016, at least 48 percent were not wearing a seat belt at the time of the crash. Research shows that seat belts reduce serious crash-related injuries and deaths by about half.

Primary Enforcement of Seat Belt Laws

State seat belt laws vary in enforcement. A primary seat belt law allows police to ticket a driver or passenger exclusively for not wearing a seat belt. A secondary law allows police to ticket motorists for not wearing a seat belt only if the driver has been pulled over for a different violation. Some states that have secondary seat belt laws permit primary enforcement for occupants under 18 years of age.

Not Drinking and Driving

Enforcing minimum legal drinking age laws and zero blood-alcohol tolerance laws for drivers under age 21 are recommended.

Drinking and driving can be deadly, especially for teens. Fewer teens are drinking and driving, but this risky behavior is still a major threat.

Teens can:

- Choose to never drink and drive
- Refuse to ride in a car with a teen driver who has been drinking
- Know and follow their state's graduated driver licensing (GDL) laws
- Follow "rules of the road" in their parent-teen driving agreement
- Wear a seat belt on every trip, no matter how short
- Obey speed limits
- Avoid using a cell phone or text while driving

(Source: "Teen Drinking and Driving," Centers for Disease Control and Prevention (CDC).)

Graduated Driver Licensing Systems

Driving is a complex skill, one that must be practiced to be learned well. A teenagers' lack of driving experience combined with risk-taking behavior puts them at a heightened risk for crashes. The need for skill-building and driving supervision for new drivers is the basis for graduated driver licensing (GDL) systems, which exist (although varied) in all U.S. states and Washington, DC. Graduated driver licensing (GDL) provides longer practice periods, limits driving under high-risk conditions for newly licensed drivers, and requires greater participation of parents as their teens learn to drive. Research suggests that the more comprehensive GDL programs are associated with reductions of 26 to 41 percent in fatal crashes and reductions of 16 to 22 percent in overall crashes among 16-year-old drivers. Knowing your state's GDL laws can help enforce the laws and, in effect, help keep you safe.

Chapter 21

The Keys to Defensive Driving

Each time you drive, you will notice that not everyone on the road is driving in a proper way or in an orderly manner; some drive aggressively, while others drive slowly and inattentively. Also, there may be drivers who make sudden turns without indicating them or who weave in and out of traffic in a dangerous manner.

You cannot control other drivers; however, learning how to drive defensively can save you from unwanted collisions and accidents caused by bad drivers.

What Is Defensive Driving?

Defensive driving is a method of safe-driving strategies that address identified hazards in a predictable manner.

Skills Required to Be a Defensive Driver

Before you take the wheel, here are some tips for you to stay in control during a hazardous event:

Be Focused

To avoid accidents, keep yourself focused while driving. Following the traffic, rules are perhaps the most basic rule and the most neglected one of all. While driving, you are expected to pay attention to road signs, road conditions, traffic signals, and speed. You should be aware of other vehicles around you while driving; this can be accomplished by checking the rear-view mirrors.

About This Chapter: "The Keys to Defensive Driving," © 2019 Omnigraphics. Reviewed July 2019.

While driving, take care not to get distracted. Avoid talking on the phone, eating, using infotainment, or getting involved in a quarrel with fellow passengers. Playing loud music can also be distracting and you may not be able to hear the sound of a horn. It will distract other drivers, too.

Be Alert

Being alert while driving allows you to react quickly to potential problems, such as a driver suddenly slamming on brakes in front of you or a driver taking a sudden turn without using a turn signal. Also, certain drugs and medications, such as over-the-counter (OTC) drugs, can cause drowsiness while driving. They affect the reaction time and judgment of a driver. Driving under fatigue is also one of the major causes of car crashes. If you feel sleepy or tired, make sure you rest before driving.

Watch Out for the Other Drivers

You should be aware of the drivers around your vehicle while driving, as this helps to drive defensively. Maintain a proper distance between you and the other drivers as this distance can prevent you from crashing during sudden braking or turning. Looking ahead while driving will help you anticipating other potentially dangerous situations, such as a pedestrian who is about to cross the road suddenly. Do not depend on others when you drive—for example, do not assume that a driver will move out of your way or allow you to merge. Plan your movements before the situation gets out of hand.

Tips for Defensive Driving

Avoiding inattentive driving and staying focused will put you in a stronger position to deal with bad drivers. Below are some tips to make your driving more effective and defensive:

- **Buckle up.** Safety is a key aspect of defensive driving; therefore, make sure you and your fellow passengers fasten all seat belts before driving. Seat belts can save you from crashing through the windshield and other actions that can cause you harm, because seat belts have a mechanism that hold you to the seat during a collision.

- **Say no to alcohol.** There is no safe amount of alcohol one can drink before driving. Impaired driving increases the risk of getting involved in a crash or collision. Moreover, drunk driving is against the law. Make sure you are not inebriated before you take the wheel.

- **Have an escape route.** The best way to avoid a crash is to drive in a position that allows you can see and be seen. Also, plan an alternate path of travel in accordance with the position of other vehicles sharing the road.

- **Drive within speed limits.** Each and every road has a speed limit; therefore, it is your responsibility to stick to that limit. Maintain the speed of your vehicle according to the permitted speed limits to avoid crashing.

- **Stay vigilant.** Staying alert throughout the ride includes watching out for other drivers' activities, and monitoring pedestrian crossings, road conditions, and road signs. Check your mirrors every time you make a turn and indicate your turn in advance. Blink your lights if you are planning to pass another vehicle. If a driver exhibits signs of aggressive driving, pull over or slow down to avoid it. If the driver is driving very aggressively, take the next exit if that is possible or try to get off the road.

- **Cut out distractions.** Driving requires complete attention, so quit using your smartphone or engaging in any other activities that may make you inattentive. If you must use for phone (for navigation, and so on), use a mounted phone holder as this will greatly help you to keep your eyes on the road.

References

1. "Defensive Driving Techniques," Drivers Ed, June 4, 2019.

2. Baumm, Alex. "Defensive Driving: What Does It Mean?" Streetdirectory, March 21, 2008.

3. "The Keys to Defensive Driving," TeensHealth, September 2016.

4. Walker, Lorrie. "You Can Keep Your Teen Drivers Safer. Here Are 7 Ways That Can Help," Safe Kids Worldwide, May 16, 2016.

Chapter 22

Graduated Driver Licensing Program

Motor vehicle crashes are the leading cause of death among teenagers. Graduated driver licensing (GDLs) systems give beginning teen drivers experience driving under lower-risk driving conditions, while allowing them time to acquire the skills, maturity, and experience necessary for full licensure. National and state-wide evaluations indicate that GDL reduces fatal crashes among newly licensed teen drivers. Importantly, the more comprehensive GDLs are associated with the greatest benefits.

As of now, all 50 states and the District of Columbia have implemented all or some of the components of a 3-stage GDLs, but specific components and timelines for progressing through the GDL stages vary from state-to-state. To reduce crash deaths and injuries involving teen drivers, state partners can assess their states' motor vehicle-related injury and crash burden among teens, their passengers, and others who share the road with teens; assess the risk and protective factors for teens in their state; develop actionable plans to reduce crashes involving teen drivers; and build and leverage partnerships with diverse stakeholders.

About This Chapter: Text in this chapter begins with excerpts from "Graduated Driver Licensing System Planning Guide," Centers for Disease Prevention and Control (CDC), December 2016; Text under the heading "How Effective Are Graduated Driver Licensing Systems?" is excerpted from "Graduated Driver Licensing System," National Highway Traffic Safety Administration (NHTSA), January 2008. Reviewed July 2019; Text under the heading "Need for More Comprehensive Graduated Driver Licensing Systems" is excerpted from "Graduated Driver Licensing System," U.S. Department of Transportation (DOT), October 26, 2015. Reviewed July 2019.

How Effective Are Graduated Driver Licensing Systems?

Evaluations clearly show the benefits of adopting GDL laws and GDL components. Florida's GDL law resulted in a 9-percent reduction in crashes for drivers who were 16 and 17 years of age. Ongoing research in Michigan and North Carolina has shown a 26 percent and 25 percent reduction, respectively, in crashes involving 16-year-old drivers. Maryland's and Texas' GDL programs showed similar success. GDL components adopted in the late 1970s and early 1980s also had positive effects. For instance, California reported a 5-percent reduction in crashes and a 10-percent reduction in traffic convictions for 16- and 17-year-old drivers, while Oregon saw a 16 percent reduction in crashes for male drivers 16 and 17 years of age. Another evaluation of Oregon's GDL system demonstrated a 29 percent decrease in crash rates for 16-year-old drivers 3 years post-GDL implementation; there was a 16-percent decrease in crash rates for 17-year-old drivers.

Nova Scotia, Canada reported a 29 percent reduction in crashes involving 16-year-old drivers, while a preliminary report from Ontario, Canada cites a 31 percent reduction in crashes for all drivers between 15 and 19 years of age. A national evaluation of GDL programs by Johns Hopkins University concluded that the most comprehensive programs are associated with reductions of about 20 percent in 16-year-old drivers' fatal crash involvement rates.

The National Highway Traffic Safety Administration (NHTSA) released an evaluation of passenger restriction laws in terms of teen crash involvements. This study evaluated passenger restriction laws in 3 states: California, Massachusetts, and Virginia. Results demonstrated that, on average, there were 740 fewer 16-year-old drivers in California involved in crashes per year as a result of the passenger restriction law. There were 173 fewer 16-year-old drivers involved in crashes per year in Massachusetts, and 454 fewer 16-year-old drivers in Virginia, both as a result of their passenger restriction laws.

How Does Graduated Driver Licensing Systems Work?

In the mid-1990s, the Insurance Institute for Highway Safety (IIHS), the National Safety Council (NSC), the National Transportation Safety Board (NTSB), and the NHTSA met to establish a national model for GDL. By establishing a national model, the various traffic safety groups sought to provide guidelines for states considering a GDL system.

The three stages of the GDL system include specific components and restrictions to introduce driving privileges gradually to beginning drivers. Novice drivers are required to demonstrate responsible driving behavior during each stage of licensing before advancing to the next level.

Each stage includes recommended components and restrictions for states to consider when implementing a GDL system. Examples of components and restrictions for each stage include:

Stage 1: Learner's Permit

- The state sets minimum age for a learner's permit at no younger than 16 years of age.

- Pass vision and knowledge tests, including rules of the road, signs, and signals

- Completion of basic driver training

- A licensed adult (who is at least 21 years of age) is required in the vehicle at all times.

- All occupants must wear seat belts.

- Teenage-passenger restrictions

- Zero alcohol while driving

- A permit is visually distinctive from other driver licenses.

- A permit driver must remain crash and conviction free for at least six months to advance to the next level.

- Parental certification of 30 to 50 practice hours

- No use of portable electronic communication and entertainment device

Stage 2: Intermediate or Provisional License

- Completion of stage 1

- The state sets minimum age of 16½ years of age.

- Pass a behind the wheel road test

- Completion of advanced driver education training (safe driving decision-making, risk education, etc.)

- All occupants must wear seat belts.

- A licensed adult is required in the vehicle from 10 p.m. until 5 a.m. (e.g., nighttime driving restriction).

- Zero alcohol while driving

- Driver improvement actions are initiated at lower point level than for regular drivers.

- Provisional license is visually distinctive from a regular license.

- Teenage-passenger restrictions: not more than one teenage passenger for the first 12 months of intermediate license. Afterward, limit the number of teenage passengers to two until the age of 18.

- The driver must remain crash and conviction free for at least 12 consecutive months to advance to the next stage.

- Supervised practice

- No use of portable electronic communication and entertainment devices

Stage 3: Full Licensure

- Completion of stage 2

- The state sets a minimum age of 18 for lifting passenger and nighttime restrictions.

- Zero alcohol while driving

Need for More Comprehensive Graduated Driver Licensing Systems

Although GDL programs have been shown to reduce fatal teen crashes, a few studies have indicated that more comprehensive GDL programs are even better at reducing teen crashes and fatalities. Such programs include higher minimum age for each stage of licensing, increased hours of supervised driving, and more driving restrictions. Another element for consideration is the enforcement of GDL systems, and the use of penalties. Comprehensive GDL systems include some or all of the following:

- Minimum age of 16 years for a learner's permit

- Mandatory holding period of at least 12 months

- Restrictions against nighttime driving between 10:00 p.m. and 5:00 a.m. (or longer)

- Limit of zero or one young passengers without adult supervision

- Minimum age of 18 years for full licensure

Driver's education programs are designed to teach teen drivers the rules of the road and to help them become safe drivers so they can acquire the necessary driving skills to prepare for and pass the road driving test and, ultimately, obtain a driver's license. Formal driver education programs exist in almost every jurisdiction in the United States. These programs generally mirror States' specific driving requirements, which assure novice drivers are being taught information relevant to State requirements. The graduated driver licensing (GDL) system, which identifies driver education as an important component, gives novice drivers experience under adult supervision and protection by gradually introducing the novice driver to more complex driving situations. In fact, multiple studies report that GDL systems reduce the number of teen crashes.

(Source: "Teen Driving," National Highway Traffic Safety Administration (NHTSA).)

Chapter 23

Safety Belts and Teens

One of the safest choices drivers and passengers can make is to buckle up. Many Americans understand the lifesaving value of the seat belt—the national use rate was at 89.6 percent in 2018. Seat belt use in passenger vehicles saved an estimated 14,955 lives in 2017. Understand the potentially fatal consequences of not wearing a seat belt, and learn what you can do to make sure you and your family are properly buckled up every time.

The Impact of Seat Belt Use

Research shows:

- Seat belts reduce serious crash-related injuries and deaths by about half
- Seat belts saved almost 15,000 lives in 2016
- Airbags provide added protection but are not a substitute for seat belts. Airbags plus seat belts provide the greatest protection for adults.

(Source: "Seat Belts: Get the Facts," Centers for Disease Control and Prevention (CDC).)

Consequences of Not Wearing a Seat Belt

Out of the 37,133 people killed in motor vehicle crashes in 2017, 47 percent were not wearing seat belts. In 2017 alone, seat belts saved an estimated 14,955 lives and could have saved an additional 2,549 people if they had been wearing seat belts.

About This Chapter: Text in this chapter begins with excerpts from "Seat Belts," National Highway Traffic Safety Administration (NHTSA), 2018; Text under the heading "Theories on Why Teens Fail to Buckle Up" is excerpted from "Increasing Teen Safety Belt Use: A Program and Literature Review," National Highway Traffic Safety Administration (NHTSA), November 2005. Reviewed July 2019; Text under the heading "Seat Belts Save Lives" is excerpted from "Seat Belts Save Lives," National Highway Traffic Safety Administration (NHTSA), March 5, 2018.

The consequences of not wearing or improperly wearing a seat belt are clear:

- Buckling up helps keep you safe and secure inside your vehicle, whereas not buckling up can result in being ejected from the vehicle in a crash, which is almost always deadly.

- Airbags are not enough to protect you; in fact, the force of an airbag can seriously injure you or even kill you if you are not buckled up.

- Improperly wearing a seat belt, such as putting the strap below your arm, puts you at risk in a crash.

- If you buckle up in the front seat of a passenger car, you can reduce your risk of:

  - Fatal injury by 45 percent

  - Moderate to critical injury by 50 percent

- If you buckle up in a light truck, you can reduce your risk of:

  - Fatal injury by 60 percent

  - Moderate to critical injury by 65 percent (National Highway Traffic Safety Administration (NHTSA), 1984)

Theories on Why Teens Fail to Buckle Up

There are many theories presented in the scientific literature on why teens have low safety belt use rates and high traffic-crash rates. Among the most frequently cited theories are the following:

- **Inexperience.** It takes time to learn how to drive a vehicle, how to drive under various circumstances and conditions, and how to react in emergency situations. Thus, the high crash involvement rate for teens. Many teens who do not wear safety belts have not been in a crash yet and have not experienced the forces and energy involved firsthand.

- **Immaturity.** Teens lack the maturity of most adults. Studies show that youth are more likely to engage in risky behaviors while driving.

- **Immortality.** Teens tend to underestimate risks of driving and crashing, and they exhibit an "optimistic bias." They do not think they will get into a crash, so they do not think they need protection if they are involved in a crash.

- **Emotionality.** This trait is sometimes termed as "raging hormones." Teen emotions affect their thinking and subsequent behavior, such as "forgetting" to wear safety belts.

- **Sensation seeking.** Many teens are adventurous and tend to seek out excitement. Not wearing a safety belt is a thrill to some.

- **Risk taking.** Many teens take greater risks in all areas of life than their adult counterparts. Because teens do not yet understand the risks involved in certain behaviors, nor the potential consequences, they often tend to act impulsively.

- **Power of friends.** Teens, especially high-school students, are greatly influenced by their peers. If peers do not wear safety belts, they probably will not either. If peers chastise them for wearing a safety belt, many teens will unbuckle it.

- **Power of parents.** Parental permissiveness or strictness could be a factor related to changing teens' behavior. Teens with parents who are persistent and monitor teen belt use, are more likely to buckle up.

- **Distractions.** There is some evidence that teens are more easily distracted while driving, especially when they have other teen passengers.

Seat Belts Save Lives

In the instant you buckle up before driving or riding in the front seat of a car or truck, you cut your risk of a fatal injury in a crash nearly in half. That is a huge return on the investment of the mere seconds it takes to put on a seat belt.

The NHTSA and law enforcement want you to wear your seat belt—every ride, every time, whether in the front seat or back, day and night—because seat belts save lives. Thanks to education and effective enforcement of state seat belt laws, an all-time record high nationwide seat belt use rate of 90 percent has been reached.

Size is not safer. If you are not buckled, being in a pickup or other large vehicle is not safer. In fact, 61 percent of pickup truck occupants who were killed in 2016 were not buckled up, compared to 42 percent of passenger car occupants who were not wearing seat belts when they were killed. Big truck or small car, seat belts are the safest bet.

Back seat? Buckle up too. Too many people wrongly believe they are safe in the back seat unrestrained. 47 percent of all front-seat passenger vehicle occupants killed in crashes in 2016 were unrestrained, but 57 percent of those killed in back seats were unrestrained. If you are in the back, you should be buckled up too.

Dangerously unbelted in rural America. People who live in rural areas might believe that their crash exposure is lower, but in 2016, there were 13,732 passenger vehicle fatalities in rural locations, compared to 9,366 fatalities in urban locations. Out of those fatalities, 49 percent of those killed in the rural locations were not wearing their seat belts, compared to 46 percent in urban locations. Whether on busy city streets or a dusty rural road, buckle up to stay safe.

In 2016 alone, seat belts saved nearly 15,000 lives. That is great news. But, if everyone involved in a crash had been wearing seat belts in 2016, we could have saved an additional 2,500 lives.

Chapter 24

What You Need to Know about Airbags

From 1987 to 2017, frontal airbags saved 50,457 lives. That is enough people to fill a major league ballpark.

Learn about the safety benefits of frontal and side airbags and why it is so important to use a seat belt—your first line of defense. Also receive important guidance on how to safely position yourself and your passengers, as well as young ones in car seats and booster seats, to prevent injury from airbags in a crash.

Protection

Airbags are supplemental protection and are designed to work best in combination with seat belts. Both frontal and side-impact airbags (SABs) are generally designed to deploy in moderate to severe crashes and may even deploy in a minor crash.

Airbags reduce the chance that your upper body or head will strike the vehicle's interior during a crash. To avoid an airbag-related injury, make sure you are properly seated and remember that airbags are designed to work with seat belts, not replace them. And children under 13 years of age should sit in the back seat.

Vehicles can be equipped with both front and SABs. Frontal airbags have been standard equipment in all passenger cars since model year 1998 and in all sport utility vehicles (SUVs), pickups, and vans since model year 1999. SABs are being offered as standard or optional equipment on many new passenger vehicles.

About This Chapter: This chapter includes text excerpted from "Air Bags," National Highway Traffic Safety Administration (NHTSA), December 17, 2016.

Airbag Deployment

Generally, when there is a moderate to severe crash, a signal is sent from the airbag system's electronic control unit to an inflator within the airbag module. An igniter in the inflator starts a chemical reaction that produces a harmless gas, which inflates the airbag within the blink of an eye—or less than 1/20th of a second. Because airbags deploy very rapidly, serious or sometimes fatal injuries can occur if the driver or passenger is too close to—or comes in direct contact with—the airbag when it first begins to deploy.

Side Airbags

Side-impact airbags inflate even more quickly since there is less space between the driver or passengers and the striking object, whether the interior of the vehicle, another vehicle, a tree, or a pole.

Frontal Airbags

Sitting as far back from the steering wheel or dashboard as possible and using seat belts help prevent drivers and passengers from being "too close" to a deploying frontal airbag. This is why rear-facing car seats should not be placed in front of an active airbag, and children under 13 years of age should be seated in the back seat.

Stay Protected: Replace Used Airbags after a Crash

Airbags can only deploy once, so make sure you replace used airbags right away after a crash, only at an authorized repair center, and before you drive the vehicle again.

Fake Airbags

You count on your airbag to protect you and others in your vehicle in the event of a crash. If your vehicle is equipped with a counterfeit airbag, there is cause for concern. Counterfeit airbags have been shown to consistently malfunction in ways that range from nondeployment to the expulsion of metal shrapnel during deployment.

Consumers whose vehicles have been in a crash and who have replaced their airbags by a repair shop that is not part of a new car dealership within the past three years or who have purchased a replacement airbag online should contact the call center established by their auto manufacturer to have their vehicle inspected at their own expense and their airbag replaced if necessary. The responsibility for replacing a counterfeit airbag will vary depending on the circumstances around the original installation of the part.

If you are concerned and have an airbag that was replaced at a repair shop recommended by your insurance company, it is recommended that you contact your insurance company. If you purchased a counterfeit airbag from eBay, it may be covered by that company's "Buyer Protection" program. Contact eBay's Customer Support center. You may also wish to contact your local consumer protection agency or the appropriate State Office of the Attorney General to determine your rights under the law, and the Better Business Bureau or the Federal Trade Commission (FTC) to file a complaint.

ON-OFF Switch

There are few circumstances under which the risk of sitting in front of an active frontal airbag outweigh the safety benefits. Under these circumstances, the NHTSA will authorize the installation of an airbag on-off switch. Authorization will be granted under the following four circumstances:

- A rear-facing infant restraint must be placed in the front seat of a vehicle because there is no rear seat or the rear seat is too small for the child restraint. (For the passenger airbag only.)

- A child under 13 years of age must ride in the front seat because the child has a condition that requires frequent medical monitoring in the front seat. (For the passenger airbag only.)

- An individual with a medical condition is safer if the frontal airbag is turned off. A written statement from a physician must accompany each request based on a medical condition unless the request is based on a medical condition for which the National Conference on Medical Indications for Airbag Deactivation recommends deactivation. (For driver and/or passenger frontal airbag as appropriate.)

- A driver must sit within a few inches of the airbag, typically because she or he is of extremely small stature (i.e., 4 feet 6 inches or less). (For the driver frontal airbag only.)

In those instances where an on-off switch is not made for a particular vehicle, the NHTSA will consider allowing an airbag to be deactivated. The approval process for deactivation is more rigorous because, while an on-off switch allows the driver or passenger frontal airbag to be turned on and off in appropriate circumstances, deactivation is not so flexible. Once deactivated, an airbag cannot be easily activated for those drivers or passengers who may need it.

ON-OFF Switch/Deactivation

Only authorized dealers and repair shops can install on-off switches and can do so only with an authorization letter from the NHTSA. If you are interested in having an airbag on-off switch installed in a vehicle you own or lease (check with the leasing company first to see if installing an on-off switch would violate the terms of your lease), you will need to:

- Before filling out the form, ensure you have read the brochure carefully: you may decide that an on-off switch is not appropriate for you.

- If you decide to request an on-off switch, you will need to certify on the request form that you have read the brochure and that you (or other drivers/passengers of your vehicle) fall into one or more of the high-risk groups for the airbag(s) for which you request a switch.

- Fill out and submit the request form to NHTSA at the following address:

  - National Highway Traffic Safety Administration

    Attention: Airbag Switch Requests

    1200 New Jersey Ave. S.E.

    Washington, DC 20590-1000

- For a faster response, write your phone number on the form (available on the NHTSA's website) and fax it to: 202-493-2833 or 202-366-6916. For questions, call the Airbag Division at 202-366-6982 or e-mail Derrick.Lewis@dot.gov.

- If the form is properly and completely filled out, the NHTSA will review the document and, if approved, will send you an authorization letter that you can take to your dealer or repair shop.

- Check with your auto dealer or repair shop to see if an on-off switch is available for your vehicle and how much the switch will cost. If a switch is available and the dealer or repair shop is willing to install it, give the authorization letter directly to the dealer or repair business. After the dealer or repair shop installs the on-off switch, they will return a form along with the authorization letter to the NHTSA, indicating that the work has been done for you.

Frequently Asked Questions about Airbags
Why Do Airbags Sometimes Fail to Deploy during a Crash?

The activation of an airbag in a crash is dependent on several important factors, including the characteristics of the crash (e.g., speed, other vehicles involved, impact direction), the individual vehicle airbag system's design strategy, and the crash sensor locations. Airbags are not intended to deploy in all crashes. There may be circumstances when an airbag does not deploy. Some possible examples follow:

- The crash conditions may be sufficiently moderate where an airbag would not be needed to protect an occupant wearing a seat belt. The seat belt may provide sufficient protection from a head or chest injury in such a crash.

- Many advanced frontal airbag systems automatically turn off the passenger airbag when the vehicle detects a small-stature passenger or child, a child in a child restraint system, or no occupant in the right front passenger seat.

- Some advanced SABs will similarly shut off the passenger side airbag system when detecting a small-stature passenger or child in the right front passenger seat who is positioned too close to the side airbag.

- In used vehicles, a possible reason for the airbag not to deploy is that the airbag may not have been replaced after a previous crash. The NHTSA recommends that airbag always be replaced after a deployment. Any airbag that fails to deploy in an injury-producing crash should be reported to the NHTSA's Office of Defects Investigation (ODI) for investigation of possible system defects and potential recall.

What Is Meant by a "Moderate to Severe" Crash?

Frontal airbags are generally designed to deploy in "moderate to severe" frontal or near-frontal crashes, which are defined as crashes that are equivalent to hitting a solid, fixed barrier at 8 to 14 mph or higher. (This would be equivalent to striking a parked car of similar size at about 16 to 28 mph or higher.)

I Just Bought a Vehicle with Advanced Frontal Airbags. Does This Mean I Can Start Putting Kids in the Front Seat Again?

No. Placing a child in the front seat, no matter what the circumstances, comes with increased risk. The NHTSA recommends that children under 13 years of age ride in the back seat in the appropriate child restraint systems for their age and size: rear-facing car seats, forward-facing car seats, booster seats, or adult seat belts.

What Should I Do When the "Pass Airbag off" (Or "Passenger Airbag Off") Indicator Light Does Not Give Me the Expected Result?

The proper operation of some advanced frontal airbag systems is highly dependent on the pressure (also known as "loading") placed on the seat bottom by the driver or passenger. Situations that add or subtract sensed weight can result in an occupant misclassification. If the indicator light does not provide the expected result, consult your owner's manual to find out how to correct the problem.

After an Advanced Frontal Airbag Deploys, Can It Be Reused?

No. Once deployed, an airbag—whether advanced frontal or another type—cannot be reused and must be replaced by an authorized service technician without delay.

Have Advanced Airbag Systems Been Tested on Child-Size Dummies?

Yes. All light vehicles (passenger cars and light-duty trucks) must meet specific safety performance criteria for dummies representing 12-month-old infants, 3-year-old toddlers, 6-year-old children, and small-stature women.

For those manufacturers electing to suppress (not deploy) an airbag for an infant or child in all crashes, the occupant-sensing devices in their advanced frontal airbag systems have been tested with child-sized dummies, representing an infant in a child safety seat and small children in and out of child safety seats, to ensure that the airbag will turn itself off.

With Advanced Frontal Airbags, Do I Still Need to Maintain 10 Inches between the Airbag Cover and My Breastbone?

Yes. To minimize the potential of any air-bag-related injury, the NHTSA still recommends keeping a 10-inch minimum between the airbag cover (in the center of the steering wheel for drivers and on the dashboard for the right front passenger), maintaining a proper seating position, and moving the seat as far back as possible (drivers should be able to comfortably reach the pedals).

How Are Advanced Frontal Airbags Different?

Frontal airbags have come a long way since they first appeared in the 1980s. Although those older airbags saved thousands of lives, they deployed the same way for every driver and passenger, causing injury and in some rare cases, death to children, small adults, and any unbelted occupants positioned too close to the airbag as it deployed. The advanced frontal airbags are better able to protect drivers and front seat passengers by using sophisticated sensing systems to determine whether, when, and how much to deploy.

Rollover Airbags

In addition to protecting drivers' or passengers' heads during a side-impact crash, some side-impact head airbags, or "curtains," can also protect occupants from injury and ejection during a rollover crash. This is important because ejection causes most injuries and fatalities in rollover crashes. Not all side-impact head airbags are designed to deploy as rollover airbags. Check with your dealer and vehicle manufacturer for the availability of side-impact head airbags that can also operate as rollover airbags.

If a rollover is detected, the side-impact head airbags are typically triggered in combination with safety belt retractors to remove slack from the safety belt and keep the occupant firmly in the seat. Most side-impact head airbags deploy downward from the overhead roof rail, very close to the side windows. In many cases the rollover sensing system can determine an imminent rollover when the roll angle is very small and all four wheels are still on the ground.

When deployed as rollover airbags, side-impact head airbags will stay inflated longer to help protect the heads of the occupants during the rollover. They also keep the occupants of the outboard seats from being thrown from the vehicle. The combination of these airbags and properly worn safety belts can significantly reduce the chance of ejection.

(Source: "Rollover Air Bags," National Highway Traffic Safety Administration (NHTSA).)

Chapter 25

Tire Safety

Safety is the top priority for anyone riding a car or any other vehicle for that matter. You should make sure you have the tools to avoid being in vehicle crashes.

Being Tirewise

The only thing between you and the road are your tires.

Tire Buyer's Frequently Asked Questions—What You Should Know and Ask

What Type of Tire Should I Buy?

This will vary by where you live and the typical weather you drive in.

- All-season tires can handle a variety of road conditions. They have some mud and snow capabilities.

- Winter tires are more effective than all-season tires in deep snow.

- Summer tires are warm-weather tires that are not designed to operate in temperatures below freezing or on snow and ice.

- All-terrain tires are mainly used on four-wheel drive vehicles. They provide a good compromise between on-road driving and off-road capability.

About This Chapter: This chapter includes text excerpted from "Tires," National Highway Traffic Safety Administration (NHTSA), December 17, 2016.

How Are Tires Rated? What Does the Tire Rating Mean?

Many tires are rated by the U.S. Government on treadwear, traction performance, and temperature resistance. It is called the "Uniform Tire Quality Grading Standards" (UTQGS), and the tire ratings are on the sidewall of every passenger vehicle tire sold in the United States.

- Treadwear grades tell you how long the tread should last. For example, tires with a grade of 200 should wear twice as long as a tire with a grade of 100. The tread on tires with the highest numeric ratings, 600 or more, should take longer to wear down.

- Traction grades tell you the tire's ability to allow a car to stop on wet pavement in a shorter distance. It is graded "AA," "A," "B" or "C," with AA being the highest rating.

- Temperature grades tell you how well the tire resists heat. It is graded "A," "B" or "C," with A being the highest rating.

How Old Is the Tire I Am Buying?

All tires have a Department of Transportation (DOT) tire identification number (TIN) on the sidewall. The last four digits represent the week and year the tire was made. The National Highway Traffic Safety Administration (NHTSA) recommends checking this date when purchasing tires, along with knowing the vehicle manufacturer's recommended tire replacement timeframe. Look on both sides of the tire. The TIN may not be on both sides.

Treadwear grades are an indication of a tire's relative wear rate. The higher the treadwear number is, the longer it should take for the tread to wear down.

A control tire is assigned a grade of 100. Other tires are compared to the control tire. For example, a tire grade of 200 should wear twice as long as the control tire.

Of current tires:

- 15 percent are rated below 200

- 25 percent are rated 201 to 300

- 32 percent are rated 301 to 400

- 20 percent are rated 401 to 500

- 6 percent are rated 501 to 600

- 2 percent are rated above 600

Traction grades are an indication of a tire's ability to stop on wet pavement. A higher graded tire should allow a car to stop on wet roads in a shorter distance than a tire with a lower grade. Traction is graded from highest to lowest as "AA," "A," "B," and "C."

Of current tires:

- 15 percent are rated "AA"

- 77 percent are rated "A"

- 7 percent are rated "B"

- Only 4 lines of tires are rated "C"

Temperature grades are an indication of a tire's resistance to heat. Sustained high temperature (for example, driving long distances in hot weather) can cause a tire to deteriorate, leading to blowouts and tread separation. From highest to lowest, a tire's resistance to heat is graded as "A," "B," or "C."

Of current tires:

- 62 percent are rated "A"

- 34 percent are rated "B"

- 4 percent are rated "C"

What Size Tires Should I Buy?

Check your owner's manual or the Tire and Loading Information Label located on the driver's side door edge or post to find the correct size for your car or truck.

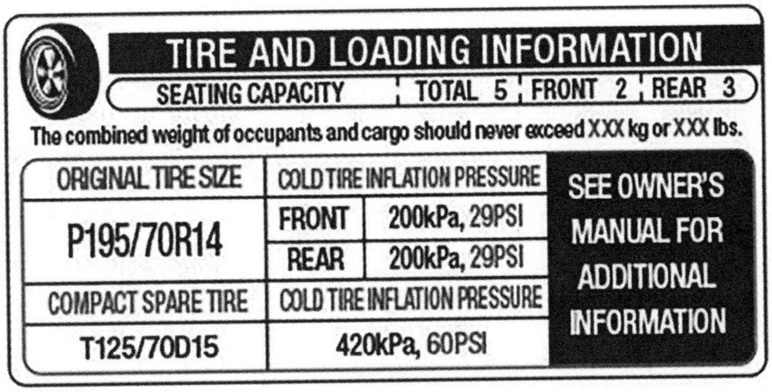

Figure 25.1. Tire and Loading Information Label

Tire Maintenance
Safety Tips

How well do you take care of your tires? Do you keep them properly inflated? Do you check if they are worn? How much do you know about basic tire maintenance and its impact on safety and fuel consumption? If you care about your safety and about saving money, it is important to understand how tires affect your vehicle's performance.

Stay Safe by Taking Care of Your Tires

- Poor tire maintenance—not having enough air in your tires and failing to rotate your tires, among other maintenance requirements—can lead to a flat tire, blowout, or the tread coming off your tire.

- In 2017, a total of 738 people died on the road in tire-related crashes.

Save Money by Taking Care of Your Tires

- Properly inflating your tires can save you as much as 11 cents per gallon on fuel. Yet, only 19 percent of consumers properly inflate their tires. That means that 4 out of 5 consumers are wasting money because of underinflated tires.

- Additional proper tire maintenance, such as rotation, balance, and alignment, can help your tires last longer, which will in turn save you money. In fact, properly inflated tires can extend the average life of a tire by 4,700 miles.

Tire Maintenance Tips for Safety and Savings
Tire Pressure

Proper tire pressure is the most important part of maintaining your tires. It affects safety, their durability, and your fuel consumption.

- Check the pressure of all tires, including your spare, at least once a month when the tires are "cold," meaning that the car has not been driven for at least three hours.

- Your tire's proper tire inflation pressure—measured in both kilopascals (kPA) and pounds per square inch (PSI or psi)—can be found on the Tire and Loading Information Label on the driver's side door edge or in your owner's manual. On new vehicles, the label will be located on the driver's side doorjamb, called a "B-pillar." If a vehicle does not have a B-pillar, then the label may be found on the rear-edge of the driver's door. If the vehicle does not have a B-pillar, and if the driver's door edge is too narrow, the label may be attached on an inward-facing surface next to the driver's seating position.

- Keep a tire pressure gauge in your vehicle. A tire can suddenly lose pressure if you drive over a pothole or bump into a curb when you park.

- Newer vehicles have tire pressure monitoring systems, but these only activate a warning when a tire is significantly underinflated. You should still conduct a monthly tire pressure check to ensure that your tires are always properly inflated.

Tire Tread

Tire tread provides the gripping action and traction that prevents your car or truck from slipping and sliding, especially when the road is icy or wet. Tires are not safe and should be replaced when the tread is worn down to 2/32 of an inch.

- Check your tire's tread at least once a month when you are checking their pressure.

- Tires have built-in treadwear indicators, which are raised sections that run in between the tire's tread. When the tread is worn down so that it is level with the tread indicator, it is time to replace your tires.

- You can also check your tread by placing a penny in the tread with Lincoln's head upside down and facing you. If you can see the top of Lincoln's head, replace your tires.

Balance and Alignment

Having your tires balanced and a wheel alignment performed by a qualified technician is important for the safety of your vehicle and to maximize the life of your tires.

- Tire balancing ensures that your wheels rotate properly and do not cause the vehicle to shake or vibrate. New tires should always be balanced when installed.

- A wheel alignment maximizes the life of your tires and prevents your car from veering to the right or left when driving on a straight, level road.

Tire Rotation

- Rotating your tires can help reduce irregular wear, which will help your tires last longer and maintain the fuel efficiency of your tires.

- Check your owner's manual for information on how frequently the tires on your vehicle should be rotated and the best pattern for rotation.

- If recommended by the vehicle manufacturer, rotate tires every 5,000 to 8,000 miles or sooner if uneven wear appears.

- For some vehicles, tire rotation is not recommended. If your front and rear tires are different sizes, you may not be able to rotate your tires. Check your owner's manual for guidance.

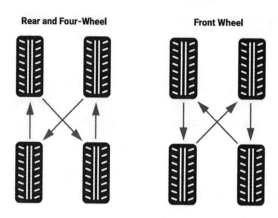

Figure 25.2. Tires Rotation Pattern

Tire Size

To maintain tire safety, purchase new tires that are the same size as the vehicle's original tires or another size recommended by the vehicle manufacturer. Check your owner's manual or the Tire and Loading Information Label located on the driver's side door edge or post to find the correct size for your car or truck. If you have any doubt about the correct size to choose, consult with the tire dealer. They can find the correct size tire for your vehicle.

Maintaining Proper Tire Pressure

Follow these tire pressure steps—they are the most important part of maintaining your tires:

- **Step 1:** Locate the recommended tire pressure on the Tire and Loading Information Labels on the driver's side door edge or post or in the owner's manual. (Remember, the correct pressure for your tires is what the vehicle manufacturer has listed, not what is listed on the tire itself.)

- **Step 2:** Check the tire pressure of all tires.

- **Step 3:** If the tire pressure is too high in any of the tires, slowly release air by gently pressing on the tire valve stem with the edge of your tire gauge until you get to the correct pressure.

- **Step 4:** If the tire pressure is too low, note the difference between the measured tire pressure and the correct tire pressure. These "missing" pounds of pressure are what you will need to add. At a service station, add the missing pounds of air pressure to each tire that is under-inflated.

- **Step 5:** Check all the tires to make sure they have the same air pressure (except in cases in which the front and rear tires are supposed to have different amounts of pressure).

Remember: The vehicle manufacturer's recommended tire inflation pressure is the proper psi (pounds per square inch) or kPa (kilopascals—the metric measure used internationally) when a tire is cold. To get an accurate tire pressure reading, you must measure tire pressure when the tires are cold or compensate for the extra pressure in warm tires.

If you have been driving your vehicle and think a tire is underinflated, fill it to the recommended cold inflation pressure indicated on your vehicle's tire information placard or certification label. While your tire may still be slightly underinflated due to the extra pressure of a warm tire, it is safer to drive with air pressure that is slightly lower than the vehicle manufacturer's recommended cold inflation pressure than to drive with a significantly underinflated tire. Since this is a temporary fix, do not forget to recheck and adjust the tire's pressure when you can obtain a cold reading.

Tire Blowouts

A tire blowout is a rapid loss of tire air pressure that can cause your vehicle to lose control. Although maintaining proper tire pressure can help you avoid blowouts, it is not always possible. Here are some tips to help you stay safe in the event of a blowout.

What Should I Do If I Have a Tire Blowout While Driving?

The goal in any blowout is to keep the vehicle balanced and controllable. Do not panic. Any overreaction—including slamming on the brakes or abruptly removing your foot from the accelerator—can result in a loss of control over the vehicle. Instead, you should take the following steps:

- Hold the steering wheel with both hands.

- Maintain your vehicle speed if possible and if it is safe to do so.

- Gradually release the accelerator.

- Correct the steering as necessary to stabilize your vehicle and regain control. Look where you want the vehicle to go and steer in that direction.

- Once your vehicle has stabilized, continue to slow down and pull off the road where and when you judge it is safe to do so.

Is There a Difference If My Front Tire Blows out as Opposed to My Rear Tire?

No matter which tire blows out—front or back—the steps for safely maintaining control of your vehicle are the same. The difference is in how you will feel it. In a front tire blowout, you will feel the force more in the vehicle's steering. In a rear blowout, you will feel it more in the seat or body of the vehicle.

Tire Pressure Monitoring System Frequently Asked Questions
How Does the Tire Pressure Monitoring System Work?

Tire pressure monitoring systems (TPMS) continuously monitor the pressure in the tires through sensors located in the tires (direct system) or through the use of wheel speed and other vehicle sensors (indirect system). The information collected by the sensors is transmitted to an onboard processor that interprets the sensor signals and warns the driver when tire pressure is below the minimum acceptable level by illuminating the TPMS symbol on your dashboard.

Does My Vehicle Have Tire Pressure Monitoring System?

All passenger cars, light trucks, and vans that are model year 2008 or newer are required to come equipped with this feature. Some model year 2006 and 2007 vehicles are also equipped with TPMS. If you own a model year 2006 or 2007 vehicle, check with your dealer or your owner's manual to determine if it comes equipped with TPMS.

What Does the Tire Pressure Monitoring System Symbol Look Like?

There are two different low tire pressure warning indicators allowed by the federal standard. One icon is the cross-section of a tire with an exclamation mark inside. The other is a top view of a car with all four tires exposed. No matter which TPMS symbol your vehicle has, it will illuminate on the vehicle dashboard when your tire pressure is significantly under-inflated.

What Does It Mean If the Tire Pressure Monitoring System Symbol Illuminates?

When the TPMS symbol appears on your dashboard, it means that at least one of your tires is significantly underinflated. You should inspect your tires and check the tire pressure as soon as possible. The symbol will extinguish after the tires are properly inflated.

What Does It Mean If the Tire Pressure Monitoring System Symbol Goes on and Off?

On cold mornings, the TPMS symbol may illuminate for a short period of time and then turn off. This is likely caused by marginally low tire pressure that dips below the warning threshold overnight but rises to an acceptable level as the tires heat up through vehicle operation or an increase in external temperatures. If the TPMS symbol goes on and off, you should inspect your tires and check your tire pressure. The lamp should not illuminate when the tires are properly inflated.

What Does It Mean If the Warning Lamp Flashes on and off and Then Remains Illuminated?

All TPMS installed on 2008 model year vehicles and beyond are required to detect and warn the driver when the system is not functioning properly. A system malfunction may be indicated by a flashing of the TPMS symbol for 60 to 90 seconds with the warning lamp remaining illuminated after the flashing sequence. The flashing sequence followed by continuous illumination of the warning lamp will repeat at each subsequent vehicle start-up until the malfunction is corrected. You should contact your vehicle dealer for a system inspection.

If the Tire Pressure Monitoring System Symbol Is On, Would Not I Have Already Noticed That My Tires Are Underinflated?

Underinflated tires are visually difficult to detect. It is recommended that you inspect tires monthly with an accurate gauge. The TPMS is not intended to be a substitute for regular tire maintenance.

Most vehicle owners can easily overlook tire aging, increasing their risk of a crash. Tire aging occurs when the rubber and other components in a tire change over time due to service, storage, and environmental conditions.

Am I at Risk?

Most of us drive our vehicles enough that the tires' treads wear out, and we replace our tires before aging becomes an issue. However, if you own or use recreational vehicles, 15-passenger vans, collector cars, any other vehicles you do not drive regularly, or if your annual mileage is low, you could be at risk.

In addition to infrequent use, exposure to sunlight and warmer climate, poor storage, and poor maintenance also contribute to tire aging. Tire aging is a greater concern in the more southern parts of the Sun Belt states.

What Can I Do?

You cannot detect tire aging simply by looking at your tires. However, there are steps you can take to extend the service life of your tires.

- Conduct monthly maintenance inspections, focusing on proper tire inflation pressure, treadwear and tire damage, along with recurring tire rotation, and balancing and alignment services.

- If your car has a tire pressure monitoring system (TPMS), pay attention to it! All passenger cars, light trucks, and vans that are model year 2008 or newer come equipped with this feature. If the TPMS symbol lights up on your dashboard, it means at least one tire is already significantly underinflated—you should take immediate action.

Should I Replace My Tires?

You should stop using tires for several reasons, including if a tire's tread is worn down to a minimum depth using the penny test, signs of physical damage (cuts, cracks, bulges, etc.), or signs of irregular wear or other damage due to underinflation or overloading. Do not use your spare as a replacement for worn tires.

Consumers are strongly encouraged to be aware of not only their tires' visual condition but also any change in how they perform. If you notice any tire performance issues, such as failing to maintain proper tire inflation pressure, noise, or vibration, consult a tire service professional.

As tires age, they are more prone to failure. Some vehicle and tire manufacturers recommend replacing tires that are 6 to 10 years old, regardless of treadwear. You can determine how old your tire is by looking on the sidewall for your DOT Tire Identification Number (TIN). The last four digits of the TIN indicate the week and year the tire was made. If the TIN reads

0308 it was made in the third week of 2008. Look on both sides of the tire. The TIN may not be on both sides.

Tires and Fuel Efficiency: It Is All about Staying "Green"

The tires you buy and how well you maintain them can significantly affect how much money you spend on fuel, as well as your vehicle's impact on the environment. Being an informed consumer and properly maintaining your tires means you can be green—and get more "green" in your wallet by reducing your vehicle emissions.

Chapter 26

Headlights and Safer Night Driving

One should be very careful when driving in the later part of the day and in the evening. As dusk sets in, careful driving becomes crucial. Driving at dusk and night requires special attention, and one should not take night drives for granted.

High-Beam Headlights

Even well-experienced drivers find it challenging to drive during low-visibility hours, and that is why headlights play a vital role in assisting you. Your headlights have two beams: the high and low beam.

Understanding when to use your high-beam lights is very important. The high beams are designed to shine at an angle that will illuminate the road up to 350 to 400 feet ahead or about twice as far as the low-beam lights. It is safest to use high-beam lights while driving on highways because low-beam lights only give you a second or two to react to a dangerous situation. Using your high-beam lights includes a few restrictions, however, that vary according to the laws of the state. High-beam lights should not be used if:

- The approaching vehicle is within 500 feet of you
- You are following a vehicle within 200 to 300 feet

Safe Usage of High-Beam Lights
Impaired Visibility in Urban Areas

If you are finding it difficult to see the road ahead of you, slow down. Turn on your high-beam lights if there are no vehicles nearby. This will help you see and avoid pedestrians and

---

About This Chapter: "Headlights and Safer Night Driving," © 2019 Omnigraphics. Reviewed July 2019.

bicyclists. Remember, you should dim your high-beam lights if an approaching vehicle is within 300 to 1,000 feet away and if you are following a vehicle within 200 to 300 feet.

Impaired Visibility in Interstate Highways

The visibility of on- and off-ramps may be difficult to see on some interstate highways. If this is the case, use your high-beam headlights to increase your range of visibility, but remember to dim your lights in accordance with state laws to ensure the safety other drivers.

Impaired Visibility in Rural Areas

Streetlights are sparse in rural areas. This could make driving more dangerous at night. Using your high-beam lights in these areas will help you avoid animals, bicyclists, and pedestrians.

When Not to Use High-Beam Lights

Do not use high-beam lights when you are driving in fog, rain, or snow because the light will pass through the fog or precipitation and get reflected back to you. Snowflakes, snowstorms, and ice crystals reflect the light even more than rain or precipitation. As a result, you would see only a wall of glare that would make your visibility even worse. Many vehicles come equipped with fog lights to enable better vision during fog.

Night Driving

The major risk factor for drivers who drive at night are reduced visibility, rush-hour risks, drowsy driving, driving under the influence of drugs or alcohol, and distracted drivers. Ways to overcome such risky factors are outlined below.

Reduced Visibility

Night-time driving is not ideal for human eyes. However, these tips can help you improve your vision and remain safe on the road:

- Get your eyes checked regularly. It helps ensure that you are able to read the roads signs at night and during the day.

- Wear anti-glare glasses as these will reduce the eye strain caused by the harsh lights of vehicles approaching you in the opposite lane.

- Clean your headlights regularly as dirt and grime may reduce their brightness and affect visibility.

- Try to look away from the lights of approaching vehicles. This will prevent you from experiencing temporary blindness.

- Clean your windshield on a regular basis as the accumulation of dirt and grime can reflect the lights from oncoming cars and make it difficult for you to see.

- Dim bright dashboard lights as they can hinder your ability to see things outside of your vehicle.

Managing Rush-Hour Risks

Staying focused and keep alert while driving during rush hours. Focusing on the following items can help keep your safe:

- Listen to your favorite music or an audio book to stay calm.

- Avoid rash driving.

- Decrease your speed.

- Do not tailgate.

- Drive using defensive-driving techniques.

- Stay alert.

- Do not use phones or indulge in other distracting behaviors.

Drowsy Driving

A study published by the National Sleep Foundation (NSF) notes that about 6,400 deaths and 50,000 serious injuries on the U.S. roads are caused by sleep-deprived drivers. Here are a few tips to avoid drowsy driving:

- Make sure you get a good night's sleep before you hit the road.

- Take turns driving if you are carpooling with others.

- Take breaks during a long drive.

- Pull over and take a nap if you feel drowsy.

- Stay away from drivers who are drifting or swerving.

Driving under the Influence of Drugs or Alcohol

It is unsafe to get in the vehicle of any driver who is under the influence of alcohol or drugs. The risk of encountering an inebriated driver increases at night, as people are leaving bars and restaurants. Never drive if you have been drinking. Call 911 immediately and report if you notice someone who seems to be impaired is driving.

Distracted Drivers

Texting, eating, or fidgeting with the radio—anything that shifts your attention away from driving—is considered a distraction. And, distractions are dangerous. The most dangerous of all of these acts is texting while driving, as this causes three types of distractions: visual, cognitive, and physical. The best way to stay safe is to put down your phone and drive.

References

1. "When Should High Beam Headlights Be Used?" Driving Tests, May 1, 2019.

2. "Night Driving," DMV.ORG, December 2, 2016.

Chapter 27

Bad-Weather Driving Tips

If you live in a part of the country that gets snow and ice, are you prepared to drive in those conditions? Planning and preventative maintenance are important year-round, but especially when it comes to winter driving.

Before You Go
Get Your Car Serviced

No one wants their car to break down in any season, but especially not in cold or snowy winter weather. Start the season off right by ensuring your vehicle is in optimal condition.

- Visit your mechanic for a tune-up and other routine maintenance.

- Have your vehicle checked thoroughly for leaks; badly worn hoses and belts; or other needed parts, repairs, and replacements.

Check for Recalls

Owners may not always know that their vehicle is under an open recall and needs to be repaired. The National Highway Traffic Safety Administration's (NHTSA) online Recalls Look-up Tool lets you enter a vehicle identification number (VIN) to quickly learn if your vehicle or one you are looking to purchase has a critical safety issue that has not been repaired.

About This Chapter: This chapter includes text excerpted from "Winter Driving Tips," National Highway Traffic Safety Administration (NHTSA), February 22, 2017.

Know Your Car

Every vehicle handles differently; this is particularly true when driving on wet, icy, or snowy roads. Take time now to learn how your vehicle handles under winter weather driving conditions.

- Before driving your vehicle, clean snow, ice, or dirt from the windows, the forward sensors, headlights, tail lights, backup camera, and other sensors around the vehicle.

- When your area gets snow, practice driving on snow-covered or icy roads—but not on the main road. Sharpen your winter weather driving skills and know how your vehicle handles in snowy conditions by practicing in an empty parking lot. See your vehicle's manual to familiarize yourself with the features on your vehicle—such as anti-lock brakes and electronic stability control—and how the features perform in slippery conditions. For example, your vehicle or pedals may pulsate when controlling traction.

- For electric and hybrid-electric vehicles, minimize the drain on the battery. If the vehicle has a thermal heating pack for the battery, plug your vehicle in whenever it is not in use. Preheat the passenger compartment before you unplug your vehicle in the morning.

- When renting a car, become familiar with the vehicle before driving it off the lot. Know the location of the hazard lights switch in case of emergency, and review the owner's manual so that you are prepared for any driving situation that may arise.

Stock Your Vehicle

Carry items in your vehicle to handle common winter driving-related tasks, such as cleaning off your windshield, as well as any supplies you might need in an emergency. Keep the following in your vehicle:

- Snow shovel, broom, and ice scraper

- Abrasive material, such as sand or kitty litter, in case your vehicle gets stuck in the snow

- Jumper cables; flashlight; and warning devices, such as flares and emergency markers

- Blankets for protection from the cold

- A cell phone with a charger, water, food, and any necessary medicine (for longer trips or when driving in lightly populated areas)

Plan Your Travel and Route

Keep yourself and others safe by planning ahead before you venture out into bad weather.

- Check the weather, road conditions, and traffic.

- Do not rush; allow plenty of time to get to your destination safely. Plan to leave early if necessary.

- Familiarize yourself with directions and maps before you go, even if you use a GPS system, and let others know your route and anticipated arrival time.

Go Over Your Vehicle Safety Checklist
Battery

When the temperature drops, so does battery power. For gasoline and diesel engines, it takes more battery power to start your vehicle in cold weather. For electric and hybrid electric vehicles, the driving range is reduced when the battery is cold, and battery systems work better after they warm up. Make sure your battery is up to the challenges of winter.

- Have your mechanic check your battery for sufficient voltage, amperage, and reserve capacity.

- Have the charging system and belts inspected.

- Replace the battery or make necessary system repairs, including simple things such as tightening the battery cable connections.

- Keep gasoline in a hybrid-electric vehicle, to support the gasoline engine.

Lights

See and be seen. Make sure all the lights on your vehicle are in working order. Check your headlights, brake lights, turn signals, emergency flashers, and interior lights. Towing a trailer? Be sure to also check your trailer brake lights and turn signals. Trailer light connection failure is a common problem and a serious safety hazard.

Cooling System

- Make sure the cooling system is in proper working order.

- Make sure you have enough coolant in your vehicle and the coolant meets the manufacturer's specifications. See your vehicle owner's manual for specific recommendations on coolant.

- Thoroughly check the cooling system for leaks or have your mechanic do it for you.

- Have the coolant tested for proper mix, proper pH (acidity), and strength of the built-in corrosion inhibitors. Over time, the rust inhibitors in antifreeze break down and become ineffective.

- Drain and replace the coolant in your vehicle as recommended by the manufacturer to remove dirt and rust particles that can clog the cooling system and cause it to fail.

Windshield
Washer Reservoir

You can go through a lot of windshield wiper fluid fairly quickly in a single snowstorm, so be prepared for whatever might come your way.

- Completely fill your vehicle's reservoir before the first snow hits.

- Use high-quality "winter" fluid with deicer and keep extra in your vehicle.

Wipers and Defrosters

Safe winter driving depends on achieving and maintaining the best visibility possible.

- Make sure your windshield wipers work; replace worn blades.

- Consider installing heavy-duty winter wipers if you live in an area that gets a lot of snow and ice.

- Check to see that your front and rear window defrosters work properly.

Floor Mats

Improperly installed floor mats in your vehicle may interfere with the operation of the accelerator or brake pedal, increasing the risk of a crash.

- Remove old floor mats before installing new mats; never stack mats.

- Use mats that are the correct size and fit for your vehicle.

- Be sure to follow the manufacturer's instructions format installation. Use available retention clips to secure the mat and prevent it from sliding forward.

- Every time the mats are removed for any reason, verify that the driver's mat is reinstalled correctly.

Tires

- If you plan to use snow tires, have them installed in the fall so you are prepared before it snows.

- Regardless of the season, inspect your tires at least once a month and before long road trips. It only takes about five minutes. If you find yourself driving under less-than-optimal road conditions this winter, you will be glad you took the time. Do not forget to check your spare tire.

- As the outside temperature drops, so does tire inflation pressure. Make sure each tire is filled to the vehicle manufacturer's recommended inflation pressure, which is listed in your owner's manual and on a placard located on the driver's side door frame. The correct pressure is not the number listed on the tire. Be sure to check tires when they are cold, which means the car has not been driven for at least three hours.

- Look closely at your tread and replace tires that have uneven wear or insufficient tread. Tread should be at least 2/32 of an inch or greater on all tires.

- Check the age of each tire. Some vehicle manufacturers recommend that tires be replaced every six years regardless of use, but check your owner's manual to find out.

Safety First
Protect Yourself and Your Loved Ones

Always wear your seat belt on every trip, every time—and ensure that everyone else in your vehicle is buckled-up in age- and size-appropriate car seats, booster seats, or seat belts.

Protect Children

- Remember that all children under 13 years of age should always ride properly buckled in the back seat.

- Make sure car seats and booster seats are properly installed and that any children riding with you are in the right car seat, booster seat, or seat belt for their age and size.

- Through thick outerwear will keep your children warm, it can interfere with the proper harness fit the child in a car seat. Choose thin, warm layers for the child instead, and place blankets or coats around the child after the harness is snug and secure for extra warmth.

- Never leave the child unattended in or around your vehicle.

- Always remember to lock your vehicle and to keep your keys out of reach when exiting so children do not play or get trapped inside.

On the Road
Stay Alert

- Keep your gas tank close to full, even with a hybrid-electric vehicle. If you get stuck in a traffic jam or in snow, you might need more fuel than you anticipated to get home or to keep warm.

- If road conditions are hazardous, avoid driving if possible. Wait until road and weather conditions improve before venturing out in your vehicle.

- On longer trips, plan enough time to stop to stretch, get something to eat, return calls or text messages, and change drivers or rest if you feel drowsy.

Avoid Risky Driving Behaviors

- Do not text or engage in any activities that may distract you while driving.

- Obey all posted speed limits, but drive even slower if necessary, for weather conditions.

- Drive sober. Alcohol and drugs impair perception, judgment, motor skills, and memory—the skills critical for safe and responsible driving.

Driving in Winter Conditions

- Drive slowly. It is harder to control or stop your vehicle on a slick or snow-covered surface. On the road, increase your following distance enough so that you will have plenty of time to stop for vehicles ahead of you.

- Know whether your vehicle has an antilock brake system and learn how to use it properly. Antilock brake systems prevent your wheels from locking up during braking. If you have antilock brakes, apply firm, continuous pressure to the brake pedal. If you do not have antilock brakes, you may need to pump your brakes if you feel your wheels starting to lock up.

Navigating around Snow Plows

- Do not crowd a snow plow or travel beside it. Snow plows travel slowly, make wide turns, stop often, overlap lanes, and exit the road frequently.

- The road behind an active snow plow is safer to drive on. If you find yourself behind a snowplow, stay behind it or use caution when passing.

- When you are driving behind a snow plow, do not follow or stop too closely. A snow-plow operator's field-of-vision is limited; if you cannot see the mirrors, the driver cannot see you. Also, the materials used to deice the road could hit your vehicle.

- Snow plows can throw up a cloud of snow that can reduce your visibility to zero in less time than you can react. Never drive into a snow cloud—it can conceal vehicles or hazards.

In an Emergency
What to Do in a Winter Emergency

If you are stopped or stalled in wintry weather, follow these safety rules:

- Stay with your car, and do not overexert yourself.

- Put bright markers on the antenna or windows, and keep the interior dome light turned on.

- To avoid asphyxiation from carbon monoxide poisoning, do not run your car for long periods of time with the windows up or in an enclosed space. If you must run your vehicle, clear the exhaust pipe of any snow and run it only sporadically—just long enough to stay warm.

Chapter 28

Drowsy Driving

Drowsy driving is a major problem in the United States. The risk, danger, and often tragic results of drowsy driving are alarming. Drowsy driving is the dangerous combination of driving and sleepiness or fatigue. This usually happens when a driver has not slept enough, but it can also happen due to untreated sleep disorders, medications, drinking alcohol, or shift work.

No one knows the exact moment when sleep comes over their body. Falling asleep at the wheel is clearly dangerous, but being sleepy affects your ability to drive safely even if you do not fall asleep. Drowsiness:

- Makes drivers less able to pay attention to the road

- Slows your reaction time if you have to brake or steer suddenly

- Affects a driver's ability to make good decisions

The Problem

According to research by the American Automobile Association (AAA) Foundation for Traffic Safety, 1 in 5 fatal crashes involves a drowsy driver, and drivers between 16 and 24 years of age are at the greatest risk for being involved in a drowsy driving crash.

Between 2010 and 2015, more than 1,300 drivers 25 years of age and younger were involved in fatal drowsy driving crashes in the United States, representing over 30 percent of all drivers in such crashes. Studies conducted in North Carolina and New York found that drivers 25 years of age and younger are overrepresented in all (fatal and nonfatal) drowsy driving crashes.

About This Chapter: Text in this chapter begins with excerpts from "Drowsy Driving: Asleep at the Wheel," Centers for Disease Control and Prevention (CDC), November 7, 2018; Text beginning with the heading "The Problem" is excerpted from "Safety Alert," National Transportation Safety Board (NTSB), February 2017.

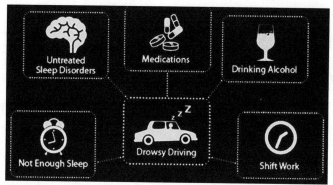

Figure 28.1. What Drowsy Driving Is *(Source: "Drowsy Driving: Asleep at the Wheel," Centers for Disease Control and Prevention (CDC).)*

Drowsy driving is the dangerous combination of driving and sleepiness or fatigue.

Survey research has found that young adults between 19 and 24 years of age are more likely to report falling asleep while driving than any other age group.

Teens need 8 to 10 hours of sleep per night, yet a study by the Centers for Disease Control and Prevention (CDC) found that more than two-thirds of high-school students get 7 hours of sleep or less on an average school night.

High-school students who reported sleeping seven or fewer hours per night were more likely to engage in high-risk behaviors, such as texting while driving, drinking and driving, and not wearing a seat belt.

What Can Young Drivers Do?

Make sleep a priority. While older adults need 7 to 9 hours of sleep per night, teens need more—8 to 10 hours for optimal health and safety.

Avoid driving during nighttime and early morning hours, when sleep typically occurs. Almost every state has graduated driver license (GDL) laws that limit when teens can drive after dark. Such laws have been shown to reduce the rates of serious crashes among young drivers.

Chapter 29

Distracted Driving

Distracted driving is driving while doing another activity that takes your attention away from driving. Distracted driving can increase the chance of a motor vehicle crash. Each day in the United States, approximately 9 people are killed and more than 1,000 injured in crashes that are reported to involve a distracted driver.

What Are the Types of Distraction?

There are three main types of distraction:

- **Visual,** taking your eyes off the road
- **Manual,** taking your hands off the wheel
- **Cognitive,** taking your mind off of driving

Distracted Driving Activities

Anything that takes your attention away from driving can be a distraction. Sending a text message, talking on a cell phone, using a navigation system, and eating while driving are a few examples of distracted driving. Any of these distractions can endanger the driver and others around them.

About This Chapter: This chapter includes text excerpted from "Distracted Driving," Centers for Disease Control and Prevention (CDC), June 9, 2017.

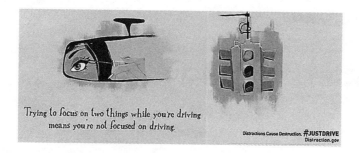

Figure 29.1. Distracted Driving *(Source: "Two Things Driving and Makeup," National Highway Traffic Safety Administration (NHTSA).)*

Texting while driving is especially dangerous because it combines all three types of distraction.

When you send or read a text message, you take your eyes off the road for about 5 seconds, long enough to cover the length of a football field while driving at 55 mph.

How Big Is the Problem of Distracted Driving?
Deaths

In 2016, 3,450 people were killed in crashes involving a distracted driver.

Injuries

In 2015, 391,000 people were injured in motor vehicle crashes involving a distracted driver.

Table 29.1. Deaths and Injuries due to Distracted Driving

	2010	2011	2012	2013	2014	2015
Distracted Driving Deaths	3,092	3,331	3,328	3,154	3,179	3,477
All Motor Vehicle Deaths	32,999	32,479	33,782	32,894	32,744	35,092
Distracted Driving Injuries	416,000	387,000	421,000	424,000	431,000	391,000
All Motor Vehicle Injuries	2,239,000	2,217,000	2,362,000	2,313,000	2,338,000	2,443,000

Who Is Most at Risk of Distracted Driving?
Young Adult and Teen Drivers

- Drivers under the age of 20 have the highest proportion of distraction-related fatal crashes.

- In 2017, 9 percent of all teen motor vehicle crash deaths involved distracted driving.
- The Centers for Disease Control and Prevention's (CDC) National Youth Risk Behavior Surveillance System (YRBSS) monitors health-risk behaviors among high-school students, including texting or emailing while driving. The YRBSS findings include:
  - In 2017, 42 percent of high-school students who drove in the past 30 days reported sending a text or email while driving.
  - Students who reported frequent texting while driving were:
    - Less likely to wear a seatbelt
    - More likely to ride with a driver who had been drinking
    - More likely to drink and drive

What Is Being Done to Prevent Distracted Driving?
States

- Many states are enacting laws—such as banning texting while driving or using graduated driver licensing (GDL) systems for teen drivers—to help raise awareness about the dangers of distracted driving and to help prevent it from occurring. However, the effectiveness of cell phone and texting laws on decreasing distracted driving-related crashes requires further study. The Insurance Institute for Highway Safety (IIHS) keeps track of distracted driving laws.
- As of March 2019, 16 states and the District of Columbia had banned drivers from hand-held phone use.
- As of March 2019, texting while driving is banned in 47 states and the District of Columbia. 2 additional states have banned texting while driving for new drivers.
- Some local governments also have bans on cell phone use and texting while driving.

Federal Government

- On September 30, 2009, President Obama issued an executive order prohibiting federal employees from texting while driving on government business or with government equipment.

- On September 17, 2010, the Federal Railroad Administration (FRA) banned cell phone and electronic device use of employees on the job.

- On October 27, 2010, the Federal Motor Carrier Safety Administration (FMCSA) enacted a ban that prohibits commercial vehicle drivers from texting while driving.

- In 2011, the FMCSA and the Pipeline and Hazardous Materials Safety Administration (PHMSA) banned all hand-held cell phone use by commercial drivers and drivers carrying hazardous materials.

- From 2010 to 2013, NHTSA evaluated the Distracted Driving Demonstration Projects. These projects increased police enforcement of distracted driving laws and increased awareness of distracted driving using radio advertisements, news stories, and similar media. After the projects were completed, observed driver cell phone use fell from 4.1 to 2.7 percent in California, 6.8 to 2.9 percent in Connecticut, 4.5 to 3.0 percent in Delaware, and 3.7 to 2.5 percent in New York.

- In 2014, NHTSA began their annual "U Drive. U Text. U Pay." campaign to raise awareness of the dangers of distracted driving.

Chapter 30

Impaired Driving

Every day, 29 people in the United States die in motor vehicle crashes that involve an alcohol-impaired driver. This is 1 death in every 50 minutes. The annual cost of alcohol-related crashes totals more than $44 billion.

How Big Is the Problem?

- In 2016, 10,497 people died in alcohol-impaired driving crashes, accounting for 28 percent of all traffic-related deaths in the United States.

- Of the 1,233 traffic deaths among children between 0 and 14 years of age in 2016, 214 (17%) involved an alcohol-impaired driver.

- In 2016, more than 1 million drivers were arrested for driving under the influence of alcohol or narcotics. That is 1 percent of the 111 million self-reported episodes of alcohol-impaired driving among U.S. adults each year.

- Drugs other than alcohol (legal and illegal) are involved in about 16 percent of motor vehicle crashes.

- Marijuana use is increasing, and 13 percent of nighttime weekend drivers have marijuana in their system.

About This chapter: This chapter includes text excerpted from "Impaired Driving: Get the Facts," Centers for Disease Control and Prevention (CDC), March 22, 2019.

- Marijuana users were about 25 percent more likely to be involved in a crash than drivers with no evidence of marijuana use; however, other factors—such as age and sex—may account for the increased crash risk among marijuana users.

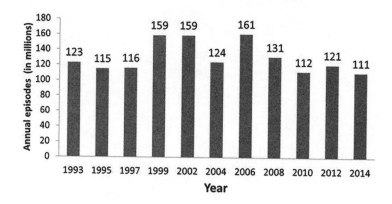

Figure 30.1. Annual Self-Reported Alcohol-Impaired Driving Episodes among U.S. Adults, 1993 to 2014. *(Source: Centers for Disease Control and Prevention (CDC). Behavioral Risk Factor Surveillance System (BRFSS), 1993 to 2014.)*

The annual estimated alcohol-impaired driving episodes were calculated using Behavioral Risk Factor Surveillance System (BRFSS) respondents' answers to this question: "During the past 30 days, how many times have you driven when you have had perhaps too much to drink?" Annual estimates per respondent were calculated by multiplying the reported episodes during the preceding 30 days by 12. These numbers were summed to obtain the annual national estimates.

Who Is Most at Risk?
Young People

- At all levels of blood alcohol concentration (BAC), the risk of being involved in a crash is greater for young people than for older people.

- Among drivers with BAC levels of 0.08 percent or higher involved in fatal crashes in 2016, nearly 3 in 10 were between 25 and 34 years of age (27%). The next 2 largest groups were of the ages 21 to 24 (26%) and 35 to 44 (22%).

Motorcyclists

- Among motorcyclists killed in fatal crashes in 2016, 25 percent had BACs of 0.08 percent or greater.

- Motorcyclists between 35 and 39 years of age have the highest percentage of deaths with BACs of 0.08 percent or greater (38% in 2016).

Drivers with Prior Driving while Impaired Convictions

- Drivers with a BAC of 0.08 percent or higher involved in fatal crashes were 4.5 times more likely to have a prior conviction for driving while intoxicated (DWI) than were drivers with no alcohol in their system. (9% and 2%, respectively.)

What Are the Effects of Blood Alcohol Concentration?

Table 30.1. Effects of Blood Alcohol Concentration

Blood Alcohol Concentration (BAC)*	Typical Effects	Predictable Effects on Driving
.02% About 2 alcoholic drinks**	Some loss of judgment, relaxation, slight body warmth, altered mood	Decline in visual functions (rapid tracking of a moving target), decline in ability to perform two tasks at the same time (divided attention)
.05% About 3 alcoholic drinks**	Exaggerated behavior, may have loss of small-muscle control (e.g., focusing your eyes), impaired judgment, usually good feeling, lowered alertness, release of inhibition	Reduced coordination, reduced ability to track moving objects, difficulty steering, reduced response to emergency driving situations
.08% About 4 alcoholic drinks**	Muscle coordination becomes poor (e.g., balance, speech, vision, reaction time, and hearing), harder to detect danger, judgment, self-control, reasoning, and memory are impaired	Concentration, short-term memory loss, speed control, reduced information processing capability (e.g., signal detection, visual search), impaired perception
.10% About 5 alcoholic drinks**	Clear deterioration of reaction time and control, slurred speech, poor coordination, and slowed thinking	Reduced ability to maintain lane position and brake appropriately

Table 30.1. Continued

Blood Alcohol Concentration (BAC)*	Typical Effects	Predictable Effects on Driving
.15% About 7 alcoholic drinks**	Far less muscle control than normal Vomiting may occur (unless this level is reached slowly or a person has developed a tolerance for alcohol) Major loss of balance	Substantial impairment in vehicle control, attention to driving task, and in necessary visual and auditory information processing

Blood alcohol concentration measurement. The number of drinks listed represents the approximate amount of alcohol that a 160-pound man would need to drink in one hour to reach the listed BAC in each category.

** Standard drink size in the United States. A standard drink is equal to 14.0 grams (0.6 ounces) of pure alcohol. Generally, this amount of pure alcohol is found in:*

- *12-ounces of beer (5% alcohol content)*

- *8-ounces of malt liquor (7% alcohol content)*

- *5-ounces of wine (12% alcohol content)*

- *1.5-ounces or a "shot" of 80-proof (40% alcohol content) distilled spirits or liquor (e.g., gin, rum, vodka, whiskey)*

How Can Deaths and Injuries from Impaired Driving Be Prevented?

Effective measures include:

- Actively enforcing existing 0.08 percent BAC laws, minimum legal drinking age laws, and zero tolerance laws for drivers younger than 21 years of age in all states

- Requiring ignition interlocks for all offenders, including first-time offenders

- Using sobriety checkpoints

- Putting health promotion efforts into practice that influence economic, organizational, policy, and school/community action

- Using community-based approaches to alcohol control and DWI prevention

- Requiring mandatory substance-abuse assessment and treatment, if needed, for DWI offenders

- Raising the unit price of alcohol by increasing taxes

What Safety Steps Can Individuals Take?

Whenever your social plans involve alcohol and/or drugs, make plans so that you do not have to drive while impaired. For example:

- Before drinking, designate a nondrinking driver when with a group.

- Do not let your friends drive impaired.

- If you have been drinking or using drugs, get a ride home, use a rideshare service, or call a taxi.

- If you are hosting a party where alcohol will be served, remind your guests to plan ahead and designate their sober driver; offer alcohol-free beverages, and make sure all guests leave with a sober driver.

Chapter 31

Drugged Driving

Drugged driving is driving a vehicle while impaired due to the intoxicating effects of drug use. It can make driving a car unsafe, just like driving after drinking alcohol. Drugged driving puts the driver, passengers, and others who share the road at serious risk.

Do You Think Driving While High Is Safe?

22 percent of teens admitted that driving while high on marijuana is common among their friends.

A survey asked how students felt about drunk driving and drugged driving. It found that:

- 68 percent of students say driving under the influence of marijuana is dangerous
- 88 percent of students say driving under the influence of alcohol is dangerous

In addition, 4.8 million young people between ages 16 and 25 admit to driving under the influence of marijuana within the past year, according to the 2017 National Survey on Drug Use and Health (NSDUH).

(Source: "Two Things Driving and Makeup," Just Think Twice, U.S. Drug Enforcement Administration (DEA).)

Why Is Drugged Driving Dangerous?

The effects of specific drugs on driving skills differ depending on how they act in the brain. For example, marijuana can slow reaction time, impair judgment of time and distance, and

---

About This Chapter: This chapter includes text excerpted from "Drugged Driving," National Institute on Drug Abuse (NIDA), March 2019.

decrease coordination. Drivers who have used cocaine or methamphetamine can be aggressive and reckless when driving. Certain kinds of prescription medicines, including benzodiazepines and opioids, can cause drowsiness, dizziness, and impair cognitive functioning (thinking and judgment). All of these effects can lead to vehicle crashes.

Research studies have shown negative effects of marijuana on drivers, including an increase in lane weaving, poor reaction time, and altered attention to the road. Use of alcohol with marijuana makes drivers more impaired, causing even more lane weaving. Some studies report that opioids can cause drowsiness and impair thinking and judgment. Other studies have found that being under the influence of opioids while driving can double your risk of having a crash.

It is difficult to determine how specific drugs affect driving because people tend to mix various substances, including alcohol. Even small amounts of some drugs can have a measurable effect. As a result, some states have zero-tolerance laws for drugged driving. This means that a person can face charges for driving under the influence (DUI) if there is any amount of drug in their blood or urine. Many states are waiting to develop laws until research can better define blood levels that indicate impairment, such as those they use with alcohol.

How Many People Take Drugs and Drive?

According to the 2017 National Survey on Drug Use and Health (NSDUH), in 2017, 21.4 million people 16 years of age or older drove under the influence of alcohol in the past year, and 12.8 million drove under the influence of illicit drugs.

The survey also showed that men are more likely than women to drive under the influence of drugs or alcohol. A higher percentage of adults between the ages of 21 and 25 drive after taking drugs or drinking than do young adults between the ages of 16 and 20 or adults 26 years of age or older.

Which Drugs Are Linked to Drugged Driving?

After alcohol, marijuana is the drug most often found in the blood of drivers involved in crashes. Tests for detecting marijuana in drivers measure the level of delta-9-tetrahydrocannabinol (THC), marijuana's mind-altering ingredient, in the blood. But, the role that marijuana plays in crashes is often unclear. THC can be detected in body fluids for days or even weeks after use, and it is often combined with alcohol. The vehicle crash risk associated with marijuana in combination with alcohol, cocaine, or benzodiazepines appears to be greater than that for each drug by itself.

Several studies have shown that drivers with THC in their blood were roughly twice as likely to be responsible for a deadly crash or be killed than drivers who had not used drugs or alcohol. However, a large NHTSA study found no significant increased crash risk traceable to marijuana after controlling for drivers' age, sex, race, and presence of alcohol. More research is needed.

Along with marijuana, prescription drugs are also commonly linked to drugged driving crashes. In 2016, 19.7 percent of drivers who drove while under the influence tested positive for some type of opioid.

How Often Does Drugged Driving Cause Crashes?

It is hard to measure how many crashes are caused by drugged driving. This is because:

- A good roadside test for drug levels in the body does not yet exist.

- Some drugs can stay in your system for days or weeks after use, making it difficult to determine when the drug was used, and therefore, how and if it can be considered impaired driving.

- Police do not usually test for drugs if drivers have reached an illegal blood alcohol level because there is already enough evidence for a DUI charge.

- Many drivers who cause crashes are found to have both drugs and alcohol or more than one drug in their system, making it hard to know which substance had a greater effect.

However, according to the Governors Highway Safety Association (GHSA), 43.6 percent of fatally injured drivers in 2016 tested positive for drugs, and over half of those drivers were positive for 2 or more drugs.

What Populations Are Especially Affected by Drugged Driving?

Teen and older adult drivers are most often affected by drugged driving. Teens are less experienced and more likely than other drivers to underestimate or not recognize dangerous situations. They are also more likely to speed and allow less distance between vehicles. When a lack of driving experience is combined with drug use, the results can be tragic. Car crashes are the leading cause of death among young people between 16 and 19 years of age.

A study of college students with access to a car found that one in six had driven under the influence of a drug other than alcohol at least once in the past year. Marijuana was the most common drug used, followed by cocaine and prescription pain relievers.

Mental decline in older adults can lead to taking a prescription drug more or less often than they should or in the wrong amount. Older adults also may not break down the drug in their system as quickly as younger people. These factors can lead to unintended intoxication while behind the wheel of a car.

Effects of Commonly Misused Drugs on Driving

Marijuana affects psychomotor skills and cognitive functions critical to driving, including vigilance, drowsiness, time and distance perception, reaction time, divided attention, lane tracking, coordination, and balance.

Opioids can cause drowsiness and can impair cognitive function.

Alcohol can reduce coordination, concentration, the ability to track moving objects, and the time it takes to respond to emergency driving situations. It can also can cause drowsiness, and it affects the driver's ability to steer and maintain their lane position.

What Steps Can People Take to Prevent Drugged Driving?

Because drugged driving puts people at a higher risk for crashes, public-health experts urge people who use drugs and alcohol to develop social strategies to prevent them from getting behind the wheel of a car while impaired. Steps people can take include:

- Offering to be a designated driver

- Appointing a designated driver to take all car keys

- Getting a ride to and from parties where there are alcohol and/or drugs

- Discussing the risks of drugged driving with friends in advance

Chapter 32

Aggressive Driving

According to the National Highway Traffic Safety Administration (NHTSA), aggressive driving occurs when "an individual commits a combination of moving traffic offenses so as to endanger other persons or property." It can also be a single deliberate act that causes another driver to react defensively.

A related and more serious behavior, road rage, can be defined as an assault by the driver or passenger(s) of one motor vehicle on those in another vehicle—using the vehicle itself or any dangerous weapon—that is triggered by an incident on the roadway. While aggressive driving is treated as a traffic violation, road rage is an intentional disregard for the safety of others and is considered to be a criminal offense.

It is estimated that more than 1,500 people are killed each year in the United States as a result of aggressive-driving incidents. And men—particularly young men between the ages of 18 and 26—are three times more likely to be aggressive drivers than women, making this behavior a significant men's health issue.

Signs of Aggressive Driving

Aggressive driving involves a range of unlawful driving behaviors such as:

- **Speeding.** This includes actions such as driving too fast for current conditions, driving above the posted speed limit, and racing.

- **Frequent lane changes.** Cutting between vehicles to move ahead of traffic, changing lanes without warning, improper passing, or any similar action can put both the driver and other motorists in danger.

About This Chapter: "Aggressive Driving," © 2019 Omnigraphics. Reviewed July 2019.

- **Running a red light or stop sign.** Ignoring a stop light, entering an intersection on yellow light, and not stopping at a stop sign are serious offenses that may cause injury to vehicle occupants and others.

- **Expressing frustration.** Condemning fellow motorists, either mentally or verbally, or making aggressive hand gestures to take out your frustration can result in violence or a crash.

- **Tailgating.** Following too closely to the vehicle ahead—especially in an aggressive manner—is one of the major causes of collisions and can result in serious injury or even death.

Other aggressive behaviors include driving recklessly; unnecessary use of the horn; excessive flashing of headlights at oncoming traffic; illegal driving on a sidewalk, median, road shoulder, or ditch; failing to yield right of way; and failing to obey traffic officers, traffic signs and control devices, or traffic laws concerning safety zones.

Avoiding Aggressive Driving

Avoid aggressive driving, as well as aggressive drivers, by following some simple measures, including:

- Drive within the posted speed limit.

- Make sure there's enough room when changing lanes or when entering traffic.

- Ensure a safe following distance between you and the vehicle ahead of you.

- Always signal before changing lanes or turning.

- To avoid traffic congestion, identify alternate routes.

- Opt for public transportation for some relief from sitting behind wheel.

- Pull over to get out of the way of an aggressive driver.

- Avoid conflict when possible. Be polite and avoid prolonged eye contact with an aggressive driver.

- Do not make offensive hand gestures, and ignore any, made at you.

- Report dangerous aggressive drivers. If you are driving, either pull over to a safe spot to call the police or ask someone with you to make the call.

References

1. "Aggressive Driving," Arizona Department of Public Safety, n.d.

2. "Road Rage & Aggressive Driving," Washington State Patrol, n.d.

3. "Aggressive Driving," Insurance Information Institute (III), n.d.

4. "Aggressive Driving," National Highway Traffic Safety Administration (NHTSA), n.d.

5. Bierma, Paige. "Road Rage: When Stress Hits the Highway," HealthDay, January 20, 2016.

Chapter 33

Speeding

Dangers of Speeding

For more than 2 decades, speeding has been involved in approximately one-third of all motor vehicle fatalities. In 2017, speeding was a contributing factor in 26 percent of all traffic fatalities.

Speed also affects your safety even when you are driving at the speed limit but too fast for road conditions, such as during bad weather, when a road is under repair, or in an area at night that is not well lit.

Speeding endangers not only the life of the speeder but all of the people on the road around them, including law enforcement officers. It is a problem that we all need to help solve.

Consequences of Speeding

Speeding is more than just breaking the law. The consequences are far-ranging:

- Greater potential for loss of vehicle control
- Reduced effectiveness of occupant protection equipment
- Increased stopping distance after the driver perceives a danger
- Increased degree of crash severity leading to more severe injuries
- Economic implications of a speed-related crash
- Increased fuel consumption/cost

About This Chapter: This chapter includes text excerpted from "Speeding," National Highway Traffic Safety Administration (NHTSA), March 8, 2018.

What Drives Speeding

Speeding is a type of aggressive driving behavior. Several factors have contributed to an overall rise in aggressive driving:

Traffic

Traffic congestion is one of the most frequently mentioned contributing factors to aggressive driving, such as speeding. Drivers may respond by using aggressive driving behaviors, including speeding, changing lanes frequently, or becoming angry at anyone who they believe impedes their progress.

Running Late

Some people drive aggressively because they have too much to do and are running late for work; school; their next meeting, lesson, or soccer game; or other appointments.

Anonymity

A motor vehicle insulates the driver from the world. Shielded from the outside environment, a driver can develop a sense of detachment, as if an observer of their surroundings, rather than a participant. This can lead to some people feeling less constrained in their behavior when they cannot be seen by others and/or when it is unlikely that they will ever again see those who witness their behavior.

Disregard for Others and for the Law

Most motorists rarely drive aggressively, and some never do. For others, episodes of aggressive driving are frequent, and for a small proportion of motorists, it is their usual driving behavior. Occasional episodes of aggressive driving—such as speeding and changing lanes abruptly—might occur in response to specific situations, such as when the driver is late for an important appointment, but is not the driver's normal behavior.

If it seems that there are more cases of rude and outrageous behavior on the road now than in the past, the observation is correct—if for no other reason than there are more drivers driving more miles on the same roads than ever before.

Dealing with Speeding and Aggressive Drivers

Speeding behavior and aggressive drivers may not only affect the speeder—it can also affect other drivers, pedestrians, and bicyclists. Here are some tips for encountering speeders on the road:

- If you are in the left lane and someone wants to pass, move over and let them by.

- Give speeding drivers plenty of space. Speeding drivers may lose control of their vehicle more easily.

- Adjust your driving accordingly. Speeding is tied to aggressive driving. If a speeding driver is tailgating you or trying to engage you in risky driving, use your judgment to safely steer your vehicle out of the way.

- Call the police if you believe a driver is following you or harassing you.

Speed Cameras

Speed cameras can reduce crashes substantially. Speed cameras, also called "photo radar" or "automated speed enforcement," records a vehicle's speed using radar or other instrumentation and takes photograph of the vehicle when it exceeds a threshold limit.

(Source: "Automated Speed-Camera Enforcement," Centers for Disease Control and Prevention (CDC).)

Chapter 34

What to Do after a Car Accident

You never know what might happen on the road, so it is best to be prepared. Keep these items in a box in your trunk:

- Battery powered radio and extra batteries

- Flashlight and extra batteries

- American Automobile Association (AAA) or roadside emergency card

- Blanket

- Booster cables (also called "jumper cables")

- Fire extinguisher (5 lb., A-B-C type)

- First aid kit

- Bottled water

- Nonperishable high energy foods, such as granola bars, energy bars, trail mix, dried fruit, raisins, and crackers

- Maps

- Shovel (in case you need to dig your car out of the snow)

- Tire repair kit and pump

- Flares

About This Chapter: Text in this chapter begins with excerpts from "Your Car's Emergency Kit," girlshealth.gov, Office on Women's Health (OWH), October 31, 2013. Reviewed July 2019; Text under the heading "How to Deal with a Car Accident" is excerpted from "How to Deal with a Car Accident," girlshealth.gov, Office on Women's Health (OWH), September 22, 2009. Reviewed July 2019.

Prepare Your Vehicle for Emergencies

Have a mechanic check the following on your vehicle prior to an emergency:

- Antifreeze levels
- Battery and ignition system
- Brakes
- Exhaust system
- Fuel and air filters
- Heater and defroster
- Lights and flashing hazard lights
- Oil
- Thermostat
- Windshield wiper equipment and washer fluid level

(Source: "Car Safety," Ready, U.S. Department of Homeland Security (DHS).)

How to Deal with a Car Accident

Right after the accident, you should:

- Stop. If you can, move your car to the side of the road or out of the way of oncoming traffic. If you cannot move your car, stay in your car with your seatbelt fastened and wait for help. Warn other drivers with flares and hazard lights.

- Help or get help for injured people.

- Call 911 or the local police department to report the accident.

- Do not say that you caused the accident.

- Exchange the following information with the other driver(s):

  - Name

  - Address

  - Phone number

  - Insurance company

  - Insurance policy number

- Driver license number
- License plate number

- Write down:
  - Description of the other car(s)—year, make, model, and color
  - Exact location of accident
  - How the accident happened
  - Phone numbers and addresses of witnesses

- Work with the police but do not admit or accept blame for the accident.

- After an accident, you and your parents or guardian should:
  - Call or see your doctor if you have any injuries
  - Report the accident to your insurance company
  - Check with your local Department of Motor Vehicles (DMV) to see if you need to report the accident
  - Contact your insurance company and/or a lawyer if you are sued
  - Contact a lawyer if you need legal advice or help making a claim or dealing with your insurance company

Chapter 35

Motorcycle Safety

The number of motorcyclists killed in crashes dropped to 5,172 in 2017, a 3 percent decrease, but motorcycle riders are still overrepresented in traffic fatalities. To keep everyone safe, it is advisable for drivers and motorcyclists to share the road and be alert, and to make themselves visible, to use DOT-compliant motorcycle helmets, and to always ride sober.

Motorist Awareness

Safe riding practices and cooperation from all road users will help reduce the number of fatalities and injuries on our nation's highways. But, it is especially important for drivers to understand the safety challenges faced by motorcyclists, such as size and visibility, and motorcycle riding practices, such as downshifting and weaving, to know how to anticipate and respond to them. By raising motorists' awareness, both drivers and riders will be safer sharing the road.

Motorcyclist Safety

If you ride a motorcycle, you already know how much fun riding can be. You understand the exhilaration of cruising the open road and the challenge of controlling a motorcycle. But, motorcycling also can be dangerous. The available data on vehicle miles traveled shows that motorcyclists are about 28 times as likely as passenger car occupants to die in a motor vehicle traffic crash. Safe motorcycling takes balance, coordination, and good judgment.

About This Chapter: This chapter includes text excerpted from "Motorcycle Safety," National Highway Traffic Safety Administration (NHTSA), 2017.

Road Ready
Make Sure You Are Properly Licensed

Driving a car and riding a motorcycle require different skills and knowledge. Although motorcycle-licensing regulations vary, all states require a motorcycle license endorsement to supplement your automobile driver's license. To receive the proper endorsement in most states, you will need to pass written and on-cycle skills tests administered by your state's licensing agency. Some states require you to take a state-sponsored rider education course. Others waive the on-cycle skills test if you have already taken and passed a state-approved course. Either way, completing a motorcycle rider education course is a good way to ensure you have the correct instruction and experience it takes to ride a motorcycle. Contact your state motor vehicle administration to find a motorcycle rider-training course near you.

Of the motorcycle riders involved in fatal crashes in 2017, 29 percent were riding without valid motorcycle licenses.

Practice Operating Your Motorcycle

Given the fact that motorcycles vary in handling and responsiveness, be sure to take the time to get accustomed to the feel of a new or unfamiliar motorcycle by riding it in a controlled area. Once you feel comfortable with your bike, you can take it into traffic. Make sure you know how to handle your motorcycle in a variety of conditions (e.g., inclement weather or encountering hazards, such as slick roads, potholes, and road debris).

Before Every Ride

Check your motorcycle's tire pressure and tread depth, hand and foot brakes, headlights and signal indicators, and fluid levels before you ride. You should also check under the motorcycle for signs of oil or gas leaks. If you are carrying cargo, you should secure and balance the load on the cycle, and adjust the suspension and tire pressure to accommodate the extra weight. If you are carrying a passenger, she or he should mount the motorcycle only after the engine has started; sit as far forward as possible, directly behind you; and keep both feet on the footrests at all times, even when the motorcycle is stopped. Remind your passenger to keep her or his legs and feet away from the muffler. Tell your passenger to hold on firmly to your waist, hips, or belt; keep movement to a minimum; and lean at the same time and in the same direction as you do. Do not let your passenger dismount the motorcycle until you say it is safe.

On the Road
Wear the Proper Protection

If you are ever in a serious motorcycle crash, the best hope you have for protecting your brain is a motorcycle helmet. Always wear a helmet meeting the U.S. Department of Transportation (DOT) Federal Motor Vehicle Safety Standard (FMVSS) 218. Look for the DOT symbol on the outside back of the helmet. Snell and American National Standard Institute (ANSI) labels located inside the helmet also show that the helmet meets the standards of those private nonprofit organizations.

Arms and legs should be completely covered when riding a motorcycle, ideally by wearing leather or heavy denim. In addition to providing protection in a crash, protective gear also helps prevent dehydration. Boots or shoes should be high enough to cover your ankles, while gloves allow for a better grip and help protect your hands in the event of a crash. Wearing brightly colored clothing with reflective material will make you more visible to other vehicle drivers.

Ride Responsibly

Experienced riders know local traffic laws, and they do not take risks. Obey traffic lights, signs, speed limits, and lane markings; ride with the flow of traffic and leave plenty of room between your bike and other vehicles; and always check behind you and signal before you change lanes. Remember to ride defensively. The majority of multi-vehicle motorcycle crashes generally are caused when other drivers simply did not see the motorcyclist. Proceed cautiously at intersections, and yield to pedestrians and other vehicles as appropriate. You can increase your visibility by applying reflective materials to your motorcycle and by keeping your motorcycle's headlights on at all times, even using high beams during the day.

Be Alcohol and Drug Free

Alcohol and drugs, including some prescribed medications, negatively affect your judgment, coordination, balance, throttle control, and ability to shift gears. These substances also impair your alertness and reduce your reaction time. Even when you are fully alert, it is impossible to predict what other vehicles or pedestrians are going to do. Therefore, make sure you are alcohol and drug free when you get on your motorcycle. Otherwise, you will be heading for trouble.

Chapter 36

Pedestrian Safety

Everyone has different preferences when it comes to transportation, but at one time or another, everyone is a pedestrian. Fortunately, there was a 1.7 percent decrease in the number of pedestrians killed in traffic crashes in 2017, totaling 5,977 deaths.

You would like to do everything you can to make sure you, your loved ones, and your neighbors can enjoy walking safely in your community. Pedestrians of all ages need guidance on maintaining safety while enjoying the benefits of walking.

> Almost half (48%) of crashes that resulted in pedestrian deaths involved alcohol for the driver or the pedestrian. One in every three (33%) of fatal pedestrian crashes involved a pedestrian with a blood alcohol concentration (BAC) of at least 0.08 grams per deciliter (g/dL) and 13 percent involved a driver with a BAC of at least 0.08 g/dL. Additionally, higher vehicle speeds increase both the likelihood of a pedestrian being struck by a car and the severity of injury.
>
> *(Source: "Pedestrian Safety," Centers for Disease Control and Prevention (CDC).)*

Know the Basics
Walking Safety Tips

- Be predictable. Follow the rules of the road, and obey signs and signals.

- Walk on sidewalks whenever they are available.

- If there is no sidewalk, walk facing traffic and as far from traffic as possible.

About This Chapter: This chapter includes text excerpted from "Pedestrian Safety," National Highway Traffic Safety Administration (NHTSA), November 5, 2018.

- Keep alert at all times; do not be distracted by electronic devices that take your eyes (and ears) off the road.

- Whenever possible, cross streets at crosswalks or intersections, where drivers expect pedestrians. Look for cars in all directions, including those turning left or right.

- If a crosswalk or intersection is not available, locate a well-lit area where you have the best view of traffic. Wait for a gap in traffic that allows enough time to cross safely; continue watching for traffic as you cross.

- Never assume a driver sees you. Make eye contact with drivers as they approach to make sure you are seen.

- Be visible at all times. Wear bright clothing during the day, and wear reflective materials or use a flashlight at night.

- Watch for cars entering and exiting driveways or for those backing up in parking lots.

- Avoid alcohol and drugs when walking; they impair your abilities and your judgment.

Driving Safety Tips

- Look out for pedestrians everywhere, at all times. Safety is a shared responsibility.

- Use extra caution when driving in hard-to-see conditions, such as nighttime or bad weather.

- Slow down, and be prepared to stop when turning or otherwise entering a crosswalk.

- Yield to pedestrians in crosswalks, and stop well back from the crosswalk to give other vehicles an opportunity to see the crossing pedestrians so they can stop too.

- Never pass vehicles stopped at a crosswalk. There may be people crossing that you cannot see.

- Never drive under the influence of alcohol and/or drugs.

- Follow the speed limit, especially around people on the street.

- Follow slower speed limits in school zones and in neighborhoods where children are present.

- Be extra cautious when backing up—pedestrians can move into your path.

Stay Safe While You Walk

- Elementary-school children are very active and impulsive. Although they are learning and growing, school-aged children 10 years of age and younger still need guidance and supervision when playing and walking near traffic.

- Strengthen your traffic safety knowledge by learning and reinforcing pedestrian safety habits.

- Walking around traffic requires the same critical thinking skills as riding a bike or driving a car: Stop, look left-right-left, be safe, and be seen.

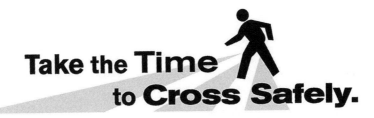

Figure 36.1. Pedestrian Safety Tip *(Source: "Pedestrian Safety Campaign," U.S. Department of Transportation (DOT).)*

Part Four
Safety at Home, School, and Work

Chapter 37

How to Be Safety Savvy

It is wonderful to be a teen. You are becoming more independent each year and are able to do new and exciting things, such as driving. But, with your new independence also comes greater responsibility and risks. For example, car crashes are the leading cause of death for teenagers in the United States. There are also safety hazards to be aware of online and out and about with friends. It is important to be aware of these risks. It is also important to know that you have the power to help keep yourself safe, whether out with friends, surfing the Internet, or even while exercising.

In Relationships

As a teen, you will have relationships with a lot of people. These relationships will probably include friendships and dating relationships. Most of the time, these relationships are fun and healthy, and they make us feel good about ourselves. Sometimes though, these relationships can be unhealthy. Unhealthy relationships can cause someone to get hurt physically or emotionally. The questions and answers below will help you understand how to spot an unhealthy relationship and how to change a bad situation.

What Is Abuse?

Some people think that their relationship is not abusive unless there is physical fighting. There are other types of abuse though. Below is a list of different types of abuse.

About This Chapter: This chapter includes text excerpted from "Safety," girlshealth.gov, Office on Women's Health (OWH), October 31, 2013. Reviewed July 2019.

Physical abuse is when a person touches your body in an unwanted or violent way. This may include hitting, kicking, pulling hair, pushing, biting, choking, or using a weapon or other item to hurt you.

Verbal/emotional abuse is when a person says something or does something that makes you afraid or feel bad about yourself. This may include yelling, name-calling, saying mean things about your family and friends, embarrassing you on purpose, telling you what to do, or threatening to hurt you or hurt themselves. Pressuring you to use drugs or alcohol is also abuse, as is keeping you from spending time with your friends and family.

Sexual abuse is any sexual contact that you do not want. You may have said "no" or may be unable to say no because the abuser has threatened you, stopped you from getting out of the situation, or has physically stopped you from leaving. This may include unwanted touching or kissing or forcing you to have sex. Sexual abuse includes date rape.

Why Are Some People Violent?

There are many reasons why a person could be violent or abusive to someone in any relationship. For example, a person who has grown up in a violent family may have learned that violence, such as hitting or verbal control, was the way to solve a problem. They may be violent because they feel bad about themselves and think that they will feel better if they make someone else feel worse. Others may get pressured by their friends to prove how strong they are. Sometimes, people have trouble controlling their anger. Yet, violence never solves problems.

Drugs and alcohol can also play a part in abusive behavior. There are some people who lose control and hurt someone after they have been drinking or taking drugs, but this is no excuse. Just because someone is under the influence of drugs and alcohol or has a bad temper does not mean that their abusive behavior is okay.

Why Do Some People Stay in Unhealthy or Violent Relationships?

Sometimes, it may be hard to get out of an abusive relationship because violent relationships often go in cycles. After a person is violent, she or he may apologize and promise never to hurt you again. They may even say that they will work on the relationship, and it may be awhile before that person acts violently again. These ups and downs can make it hard to leave a relationship.

It is also hard to leave someone you care about. You may be scared or ashamed to admit that you are in an abusive relationship, or you may simply be scared to be alone without that person. You may be afraid that no one will believe you, or that your friend or partner will hurt you more if you tell someone. Whatever the reasons, leaving an unhealthy relationship is hard, but it is something you should do.

Why Should I Leave?

Abusive relationships are very unhealthy for you. You can have trouble sleeping or have headaches or stomach aches. You might feel depressed, sad, anxious, or nervous, and you may even loose or gain weight. You may also blame yourself, feel guilty, and have trouble trusting other people in your life. Staying in an abusive relationship can hurt your self-esteem and make it hard for you to believe in yourself. If you are being physically abused, you can be in pain and may suffer permanent damage. You should definitely leave the relationship if you are getting hurt or if you are being threatened with physical harm in any way.

The most important reason to leave an unhealthy relationship is because you deserve to be in a relationship that is healthy and fun.

What Else Do I Need to Know?

At least 1 in 10 teens experience physical violence in their relationships. Even if you have not experienced physical, sexual, or verbal and emotional abuse, one of your friends may be in an unhealthy relationship with another friend or dating partner. If you are in an unhealthy relationship, or if your friend is, it is important to get help right away before someone gets hurt.

Having Fun and Staying Safe

As a teen, your family may give you more responsibilities and the chance to spend more time with your friends. This extra time with your friends may put you in new or different social situations and places. With your parents not around as much, you are making more choices for yourself and will need to keep yourself safe. If you forget about your safety, your fun can quickly turn into danger.

How Do I Keep Myself Safe at a Party?

New social settings, such as parties, are a fun way for you to spend time with your friends. Most of the time parties are safe, but sometimes things can happen that can make a party a dangerous place to be. It is important to know what to do if a party gets out of control and how to keep yourself safe.

- Never walk away with strangers.

- Never be alone with someone who has been drinking or taking drugs.

- Do not drink alcohol or do drugs.

- Tell your parents and friends where you are going.

- Never get in a car with someone who has been drinking or doing drugs.

What If Someone Offers Me Alcohol or Drugs?

You are more likely to be offered alcohol or drugs by a friend than a stranger. It is okay to say no to friends. Many people are focused on themselves, so they will not be as worried about what you are doing as you may think. Below are eight great ways to turn down an offer.

- No thanks.

- I am not into that.

- Alcohol is not my thing.

- I do not feel like it—do you have any soda?

- I am okay. Thanks.

- No, I am training for _____.

- No, I am on the _____ team, so I do not want to risk it.

- No. I gotta go soon.

You can set an example for others by staying away from drugs and alcohol. You might be worried about not being "cool" if you do not try drugs or alcohol, but you can start a different, more real kind of "cool" by being looked up to as someone who makes confident choices.

How Can I Make a Safety Plan for Different Social Situations?

No matter what the situation is, you can create a plan to help keep yourself safe. Read the following list, and create your safety plan right now.

- Tell your parents where you are going, who you will be with, and when you will be back. This may sound lame, but you will be safer for doing so.

- Carry money, a phone card, or a cell phone in case you need to make an emergency phone call. Do not forget to keep emergency numbers and the phone number of a taxi service in your wallet or backpack, or program them into your cell phone.

- Stay in well-lit public places.

- Stick with another person or a group of your friends.

- Be aware that drugs used for sexual assault often are slipped into drinks. Open your own drinks, and keep your own drink with you at all times. Try to avoid strangers. If you talk to them, do not share information about yourself.

- Use code words on the phone that you and your family decide on ahead of time. If you are in trouble, say the code word so that your family member knows you cannot talk openly and need to be picked up right away.

What Do I Do If I Am Walking in a Neighborhood I Do Not Know Well?

There are certain things that you can do to keep yourself safe until you are near home.

- Walk with another person whenever possible.

- Walk on the sidewalk of main streets, and stay where it is well-lit.

- Do not walk with headphones so that you can hear what is going on around you.

- If you think that you are being followed, cross the street to see if the person does the same. Do not be afraid to start running if you need to—do not wait until the person is very close to you to do this. Go to the nearest store, restaurant, or police station.

- Walk quickly and confidently.

- If someone grabs your purse or bag, just let go. Do not struggle with them to try to get it back. If you fight, you risk getting hurt. Money and other stuff can be replaced—your safety is the most important thing. Run in the opposite direction of the person and go to the nearest police station or store to call for help.

- If you are in trouble, yell. This will get the attention of the people around you.

What Do I Do If I Am out and Someone That I Do not Know Comes up to Me?

When you were younger, your parents probably taught you never to talk to strangers. This is a good rule for children, but in your teenage years, it does not always seem to fit. There are lots of times when you might need to talk to someone that you do not know. Most strangers are nice people, but it is important that you do not trust everyone that you meet right away.

Know the warning signs and how to protect yourself:

- **Be aware** of anyone in a car who stops to talk to you or ask you for directions if you are walking down the street, even if you are in a familiar neighborhood. Try to keep your distance from the car and never offer to get in the car—even if the stranger is going in the same direction that you are headed or if the stranger says there is an emergency.

- **Be assertive.** If a person that you do not know comes up to you to start a conversation, you do not have to talk to them if you do not feel comfortable. Do not be afraid to sound rude if someone keeps bothering you. Stay calm, and firmly say "no."

- **Be street smart.** Not all dangerous strangers are rude or forceful right away when you first meet them. It is important that you are aware of strangers, both men and women, who seem nice—the ones who make conversation easily and get important information about you without you even realizing it. Remember that you do not have to share any information. If a stranger tells you where she or he lives, it does not mean that you have to tell her or him where you live.

- **Be careful who you trust.** Keep your distance from a new person until you have had the chance to get to know her or him. Do not trust someone who follows you around or will not leave you alone if you ask them to. You can make up code words with your family that they will use if there is an emergency at home. This way, if a stranger comes up to you and says that there is an emergency and that you need to leave with them, you can ask for the code words that only you and your parents know. If you are worried or nervous, you can go to police officers or security guards with name tags and badges. You will also find people who may be able to help you at information desks and customer service desks at public places, such as the mall; restaurant or store managers may also be able to help you.

- **Be prepared.** Check out self-defense classes in your town. Your local police department or school might offer classes that can teach you how to protect yourself and how to handle uncomfortable situations. Thinking ahead and planning for your safety is a way to feel powerful and confident.

You do not have to be afraid every time you leave the house. But, it is important that you take some responsibility for your own safety. Trust your instincts, pay attention to what is going on around you, and protect yourself. Remember, being safe will not take away from your fun. Being safe will make sure that you can keep having it.

On the Road

It is late, you are tired, and all you want to do is get in the car so you can go home. But, what if the driver is drunk? The answer is simple—do not get into the car. If the driver is drunk, it is going to be a long time before it is safe for her or him to drive. To protect yourself, you must find another way home. Ask someone else to drive, call your parents/guardians, call another friend, or take a cab. Some cities have safe ride programs, where you can call a number and get a free ride home. Ask your parents/guardians for help finding out if your city has a safe ride program before you need it.

If the driver is a parent/guardian or another adult, it may be hard for you to say that you will not get in the car. Do not be afraid to ask if the person has been drinking. She or he may be surprised or offended by the question, but it is your right to have a safe ride home. If your parent/guardian is the one who is driving drunk, talk to another adult you trust for help in the future.

Some of the same advice applies to taking rides from a driver who is over-tired. Ask someone else to drive or suggest that the driver stop to rest before continuing.

You may also be driving with friends or family members who recently got their driver's licenses. New drivers may be too willing to take risks on the road, or may be careless and unsafe. Take notice, and do not be afraid to speak up for your safety or to find a different way to get to where you are going.

Safe Driving Tips

- Always wear your seat belt. Make sure your passengers buckle up too.

- Keep your doors locked at all times.

- Never drive with more people in your car than you have seat belts for.

- Try not to drive with more than one passenger. The more passengers in your car, the more likely you are to get in an accident. More passengers mean more distractions.

- Do not drink and drive.

- Do not drive if you are sleepy.

- Do not talk on the phone, text, put on makeup, brush your hair, or eat while driving.

- Do not play with the radio while you are driving. Wait until you are stopped or ask your passenger to change the station or adjust the volume.

- Always be aware of your surroundings. Be on the lookout for motorcycles, people crossing the street, and bikers.

- Do not be an aggressive driver. Aggressive drivers speed, follow too closely, or weave in and out of lanes.

- Do be a defensive driver. Defensive drivers drive the speed limit, follow at a safe distance, and are alert and aware of their surroundings.

Keep Your Car in Good Working Order

You may think of a car as simply a way to get from point A to point B, but cars need regular care to work properly. Make sure to review these items in your car regularly to keep your car safe and in good condition. Routine maintenance can save you money and keep you safe.

- **Remember to change the oil.** Your car's oil should be changed every 3,000 to 5,000 miles. The oil level should be checked every few weeks, or monthly.

- **Pay attention to the transmission.** Trouble changing gears could mean a problem with the transmission. Have your transmission checked when you get an oil change; low fluid could mean you have a leak.

- **Be sure your car has coolant.** Coolant is a mixture of antifreeze and water that keeps the temperature of your engine low.

- **Check your tires.** Learn how to check the pressure in your tires, and keep them properly inflated. Overinflated and underinflated tires can be dangerous, and they also waste gas. Also, be sure your tires have enough tread. A penny is often the simplest way to check tire tread—tick a penny into a groove with Lincoln's head pointing down. If the tread is lower than Lincoln's hair, your tire level is unsafe.

- **Brake safety.** If you hear a whining, screeching, or grinding sound, or if you feel pulling or softness when you press the brakes, get your car looked at by a mechanic right away.

- **Check belts for wear and tear.** If you are driving an older car, make sure the seat belts are not frayed or damaged in any way. You want to be sure they are in working condition in case of an accident.

- **Do not forget to fill up.** It may sound obvious, but do not forget to keep gas in your car. Fill up when your car reaches one-quarter of a tank to keep your car in good working condition and so that you never run out while on the road.

Staying Safe on Public Transportation

Keep these safety tips in mind when riding on a bus or on the subway.

- **Stay seated on all kinds of buses.** Riding the school bus or a public bus can be a lot of fun, especially when you are with your friends, but it is important to stay seated. Leaning over the back of a seat to talk to your friend is distracting to the driver and dangerous in case of an accident. Always stay seated on a bus.

- **If your bus has a seat belt, use it.** Some school buses and most public buses do not have seat belts. However, if your bus does have one, buckle up. It will keep you safer in case there is an accident.

- **Watch out when exiting the bus.** When you get off the school bus or a public bus, take five giant steps out of the door. Then pause for a moment and look around to make sure it is safe to cross the street. If you are exiting a school bus, the driver should wait for you to cross the road, if needed. Never cross in front of a public bus. Wait until the bus has pulled away and you can see when traffic has cleared so you can safely cross the street.

- **Pay attention on the platform.** If you ride the subway, do not ever play on the subway platform. It would be easy to fall onto the tracks.

At Home

Many people feel the safest at home. Even at home, though, there are some important steps you should take to protect yourself.

- Always know who is at the door before opening it. If you are home by yourself and do not recognize the person, do not open the door.

- If you are home by yourself, do not let others know. Only your parents should know that you are alone.

- If you are home by yourself and someone calls asking for your parents, tell him or her that your parents are not available and offer to take a message.

- If a stranger wants to use your phone, tell him or her you cannot help.

- If you arrive home and find that your home has been broken into, do not go in. Leave right away and call the police.

- Keep your doors and windows locked at all times.

- Keep emergency numbers for police, fire, and poison control handy.

- If your house has an alarm system, make sure your parents show you how to use it.

In School

School should be a place where we feel safe from harm. Many students attend schools that are very safe and comfortable places to learn. There still may be a time when you feel unsafe because other students use violence, or bullying, to harm you. Sexual harassment can also make you feel unsafe. Someone is sexually harassing you if she or he says or does anything sexual to make you feel uncomfortable. Some ways this can happen include:

- Making sexual comments or jokes

- Touching you in a sexual way

- Blocking your way or cornering you in a sexual way

- Forcing you to kiss her or him, or do other things that make you uncomfortable

While it is very rare for an adult at school to harass or threaten students in a sexual way, you should let a parent or guardian know right away if an adult at school makes you feel uncomfortable. You have the right to feel safe and to be respected by your classmates and adults at school. If you ever feel afraid or threatened, tell a teacher, school counselor, parent/guardian, or other adult you can trust.

Violence

Have you ever felt unsafe at school? Have you ever been afraid to go to school? If someone has threatened you, tell a parent/guardian or teacher immediately. Some students are starting to take safety into their own hands. It is a student-led effort that helps young people take responsibility for their own school community.

Chapter 38

Gun Safety

A gun is a weapon consisting of a metal tube, with mechanical attachments, from which projectiles are shot by the force of an explosive. The most important point to remember while handling a gun is that guns are not toys and they can be very dangerous if handled incorrectly. They could hurt or even kill someone.

To safely handle a gun and keep you and your family members protected, follow the rules described below.

Gun Safety Rules

- Treat your gun as if it is loaded.
- Keep your firearm pointed toward the safest possible direction.
- Keep your finger away from the trigger unless you intend to fire the gun.
- Never store your gun loaded.
- Wear safety goggles and ear protection when firing a gun.
- Know your target and the space surrounding and beyond it.
- Never point a gun at anyone, even for fun.
- Make sure you use child safety locks and store the ammunition away from the firearm.
- Make sure that you are familiar with the gun's mechanisms and learn how to handle it safely.

About This Chapter: "Gun Safety," © 2019 Omnigraphics. Reviewed July 2019.

- Obey all federal, local, and state laws regarding possession, use, storage, and disposition or sale of firearms.

Rules for Safe Gun Storage

If your parents or family members own a gun, make sure that they follow these rules for safe gun storage.

- Secure your firearm in a place that is accessible only by adults.

- Keep all guns away from children and inexperienced adults.

- Always store the gun with the safety on and make sure that it is unloaded.

- Keep all guns clean, dry, and oiled while in storage.

- Make sure that all guns and bullets are stored in a cool, dry place.

- Always keep the keys to gun safes and gun locks hidden.

Gun Safety and Depression

The American Academy of Pediatrics (AAP) notes that adolescence is an especially vulnerable stage of life during which teenagers are struggling to develop their identity, autonomy, and independence.

Depression can act as a catalyst and usher in suicidal thoughts.

It is crucial that a parent take responsibility for keeping firearms and bullets separate from each other and in a place accessible only to adults. It is also important that firearms are not loaded and are properly locked while in storage. Make sure that all guns and bullets are away from teens:

- Who are likely to experience depression

- Who may be abusive to other people

- Who may be abusing drugs or alcohol

If you feel depressed, seek help.

- Talk to your parent, teacher, school counselor, coach, or another trusted adult in your family.

- Get treated, as this will likely improve your situation.

- Call the suicide crisis line (800-273-8255) or call 911. These experts will help you get through your toughest moment.

Research indicates that about 40 percent of teens commit suicide using guns. Teens who are angry or depressed are more likely to harm or hurt themselves if they have a gun. It is advisable that parents do not have a gun in the home if a child or teen is depressed, troubled, or having suicidal thoughts.

Gun Safety Outside the Home

Teens sometimes carry a gun outside the home. They may carry it for protection, to earn attention from others, or to hurt themselves and others. If you discover that someone is carrying a gun:

- Leave the place immediately and quietly.

If you discover a gun outside

- Do not touch the gun, even if it looks like a toy.
- Make sure to inform a trusted adult or call 911.

Staying Safe While Using a Gun for Recreational Purposes

If you are using a gun for recreational purposes, make sure that you follow these rules:

- Do not handle a gun when you are alone.
- Use a gun only when accompanied by a responsible parent or other adult.
- Always assume that the gun is loaded.
- Do not point a gun at anyone or anything, even if it is not loaded.

Top Things to Know to Keep Yourself Safe

- Advise your parents not to keep guns at home and, if they have them, ask them to keep the guns unloaded and locked up. Only your parent or a responsible, trusted adult should know how to open the gun safe.
- Do not hang around with people who carry guns and do not go to places where there are guns.

- If you are depressed or having thoughts of killing yourself or hurting others, get help right away.

To avoid gun injuries and accidents, it is best not to have a gun at home and to avoid homes in which guns are kept.

References

1. "Gun Safety," TeensHealth, April 19, 2018.

2. "Gun Safety," North Carolina Department of Public Safety (NCDPS), February 26, 2016.

3. "Gun Safety," New York Secure Ammunition and Firearms Enforcement (NYSAFE), April 5, 2013.

4. "Gun Safety," Family Doctor, September 7, 2017.

Chapter 39

School and School Bus Safety

While our nation's schools are expected to be, and usually are, safe havens for learning, unintentional injuries and even violence can occur, disrupting the educational process and negatively affecting the school and surrounding community.

Get to School Safely
School Buses

School buses are the safest way for you to travel to and from school, but there are dangers when you are boarding and leaving the bus. Over the last decade, nearly two-thirds of school-age pedestrians fatally injured in school transportation-related crashes were struck by school buses or other vehicles when the children were getting on or off a school bus. You should:

- Wait five giant steps away from the road, and when the school bus arrives, wait until the driver says to board.

- Quickly find a seat after boarding, sit facing the front, and do as the bus driver says.

- Before you get to your stop, put your phone away.

- Before getting off the bus, look out the door—left, right, and then left again—for approaching vehicles.

About This Chapter: Text in this chapter begins with excerpts from "Safe Youth, Safe Schools," Centers for Disease Control and Prevention (CDC), August 4, 2017; Text under the heading "Get to School Safely" is excerpted from "Back-to-School Safety," National Highway Traffic Safety Administration (NHTSA), August 14, 2018; Text under the heading "Playground Safety" is excerpted from "Playground Safety," Centers for Disease Control and Prevention (CDC), May 2, 2016.

- Once off the bus, take five giant steps away from the school bus.

- Before crossing the street in front of the bus, go to the edge of the bus, look left-right-left to make sure no traffic is coming, and wait for the driver to signal it is safe to cross.

Walking

Walking to school is great exercise, but make sure you walk safely. You should always:

- Watch the road, not your phone.

- Walk on the sidewalk or, if there is none, walk facing traffic.

- Never play, push, or shove others when you walk around traffic.

- When crossing the street, cross at a corner or marked crosswalk.

- Stop and look left-right-left for vehicles, motorcycles, and bicyclists. Wait to cross after traffic has passed.

- Make sure to push the pedestrian button, and wait for pedestrian crossing signals, if available.

Biking

Biking is a fun, healthy way to get to and from school too. You should always:

- Wear a properly fitted helmet, and make sure to buckle the chin strap.

- Always ride in the same direction as traffic, and stop at all stop signs and signals.

- Plan to use routes that offer bike lanes when possible and that have lower traffic volume and speeds.

- Only ride on the sidewalk when necessary; ride in the same direction as traffic, be careful of pedestrians, and use caution when crossing streets.

- Never use headphones or cell phones while riding.

Vehicles

Make sure there is a safe driver behind the wheel. Every ride begins with everyone wearing seat belts, using a booster, or being properly secured in an appropriate car seat. Every child should ride in the back seat; children in the front seat are 40 percent more likely to be injured in crashes.

Playground Safety

Each year in the United States, emergency departments (EDs) treat more than 200,000 children 14 years of age and younger for playground-related injuries. More than 20,000 of these children are treated for a traumatic brain injury (TBI), including concussion.

Injury Risk Factors
All Emergency Department-Treated, Playground-Related Injuries

- While all children who use playgrounds are at risk for injury, boys sustain ED-treated injuries (55%) slightly more often than girls (45%).

- Children between the ages of 5 and 9 have higher rates of ED visits for playground injuries than any other age group. Most of these injuries occur at school. On public playgrounds, more injuries occur on monkey bars and climbing equipment than on any other equipment.

- Playgrounds that are well-maintained have fewer risks to children from rusty or broken equipment.

Playground-Related Traumatic Brain Injuries

- Boys more often sustain playground-related TBIs compared to girls.

- Most children who are treated for playground-related TBIs are 5 to 9 years of age.

- Playground-related TBIs varied by age group and equipment type:

  - 0- to 4-year-olds are often injured on swings and slides.

  - 5- to 9-year-olds are often injured on swings, monkey bars, and climbing equipment.

  - 10- to 14-year-olds are often injured on swings, monkey bars, and climbing equipment.

  - 5- to 14-year-olds sustain TBIs more frequently at school.

What Can Be Done?

Take steps to ensure your safety:

- Check the playgrounds if it has soft material under them such as wood chips, sand, or mulch.

- Read playground signs, and use playground equipment that is right for your age.

- Make sure there are guardrails in good condition to help prevent falls.

- Look out for things in the play area that can trip you, such as tree stumps or rocks.

Chapter 40

Fire Safety and Escape Planning

In just two minutes, a fire can become life-threatening. In five minutes, a residence can be engulfed in flames.

- **Fire is fast.** In less than 30 seconds, a small flame can turn into a major fire. It only takes minutes for thick black smoke to fill a house or for it to be engulfed in flames.

- **Fire is hot.** Heat is more threatening than flames. Room temperatures in a fire can be 100 degrees at floor level and rise to 600 degrees at eye level. Inhaling this super-hot air will scorch your lungs and melt clothes to your skin.

- **Fire is dark.** Fire starts bright, but it quickly produces black smoke and complete darkness.

- **Fire is deadly.** Smoke and toxic gases kill more people than flames do. Fire produces poisonous gases that make you disoriented and drowsy. Asphyxiation is the leading cause of fire deaths, exceeding burns by a three-to-one ratio.

Before a Fire
Create and Practice a Fire Escape Plan

In the event of a fire, remember that every second counts, so you and your family must always be prepared. Escape plans help you get out of your home quickly.

About This Chapter: This chapter includes text excerpted from "Home Fires," Ready, U.S. Department of Homeland Security (DHS), October 7, 2011. Reviewed July 2019.

Twice each year, practice your home fire escape plan. Some tips to consider when preparing this plan include:

- Find two ways to get out of each room in the event the primary way is blocked by fire or smoke.

- A secondary route might be a window onto a neighboring roof or a collapsible ladder for escape from upper story windows.

- Make sure that windows are not stuck, screens can be taken out quickly, and that security bars can be properly opened.

- Practice feeling your way out of the house in the dark or with your eyes closed.

- Teach children not to hide from firefighters.

Smoke Alarms

A working smoke alarm significantly increases your chances of surviving a deadly home fire.

- Install both ionization and photoelectric smoke alarms, or dual sensor smoke alarms, which contain both ionization and photoelectric smoke sensors.

- Test batteries monthly.

- Replace batteries in battery-powered and hard-wired smoke alarms at least once a year (except nonreplaceable 10-year lithium batteries).

- Install smoke alarms on every level of your home, including the basement, both inside and outside of sleeping areas.

- Replace the entire smoke alarm unit every 8 to 10 years or according to the manufacturer's instructions.

- Never disable a smoke alarm while cooking—it can be a deadly mistake.

Smoke Alarm Safety for People with Access or Functional Needs

- Audible alarms for visually impaired people should pause with a small window of silence between each successive cycle so that they can listen to instructions or voices of others.

- Smoke alarms with a vibrating pad or flashing light are available for the hearing impaired. Contact your local fire department for information about obtaining a flashing or vibrating smoke alarm.

- Smoke alarms with a strobe light outside the home to catch the attention of neighbors, and emergency call systems for summoning help, are also available.

More Fire Safety Tips

- Make digital copies of valuable documents and records, such as birth certificates.

- Sleep with your door closed.

- Contact your local fire department for information on training on the proper use and maintenance of fire extinguishers.

- Consider installing an automatic fire sprinkler system in your residence.

During a Fire

- Crawl low under any smoke to your exit—heavy smoke and poisonous gases collect first along the ceiling.

- Before opening a door, feel the doorknob and door. If either is hot, or if there is smoke coming around the door, leave the door closed and use your second way out.

- If you open a door, open it slowly. Be ready to shut it quickly if heavy smoke or fire is present.

- If you cannot get to someone needing assistance, leave the home and call 911 or the fire department. Tell the emergency operator where the person is located.

- If pets are trapped inside your home, tell firefighters right away.

- If you cannot get out, close the door and cover vents and cracks around doors with cloth or tape to keep smoke out. Call 911 or your fire department. Say where you are, and signal for help at the window with a light-colored cloth or a flashlight.

- If your clothes catch fire, stop, drop, and roll—stop immediately, drop to the ground, and cover your face with your hands. Roll over and over or back and forth until the fire is out. If you or someone else cannot stop, drop, and roll, smother the flames with a blanket or towel. Use cool water to treat the burn immediately for three to five minutes. Cover with a clean, dry cloth. Get medical help right away by calling 911 or the fire department.

Fire Escape Planning for Older Adults and People with Access or Functional Needs

- Live near an exit. You will be safest on the ground floor if you live in an apartment building. If you live in a multi-story home, arrange to sleep on the ground floor, and near an exit.

- If someone uses a walker or wheelchair, check all exits to be sure they can get through the doorways.

- Make any necessary accommodations, such as providing exit ramps and widening doorways, to facilitate an emergency escape.

- Speak to your family members, building manager, or neighbors about your fire safety plan and practice it with them.

- Contact the local fire department's nonemergency line and explain any special needs. Ask emergency providers to keep this special needs information on file.

- Keep a phone near your bed, and be ready to call 911 or your local emergency number if a fire occurs.

After a Fire

The following checklist serves as a quick reference and guide for you to follow after a fire strikes.

- Contact your local disaster relief service, such as the Red Cross, if you need temporary housing, food, and medicines.

- If you are insured, contact your insurance company for detailed instructions on protecting the property, conducting inventory, and contacting fire damage restoration companies. If you are not insured, try contacting private organizations for aid and assistance.

- Check with the fire department to make sure your residence is safe to enter. Be watchful of any structural damage caused by the fire.

- The fire department should see that utilities are either safe to use or are disconnected before they leave the site. Do not attempt to reconnect utilities yourself.

- Conduct an inventory of damaged property and items. Do not throw away any damaged goods until an inventory is made.

- Try to locate valuable documents and records.

- Begin saving receipts for any money you spend related to fire loss. The receipts may be needed later by the insurance company and for verifying losses claimed on income tax.

- Notify the mortgage company of the fire.

Prevent Home Fires

Home fires are preventable. The following are simple steps that each of us can take to prevent a tragedy.

Cooking

- Stay in the kitchen when you are frying, grilling, or broiling food. If you leave the kitchen for even a short period of time, turn off the stove.

- Wear short, close-fitting or tightly rolled sleeves when cooking.

- Keep children away from cooking areas by enforcing a "kid-free zone" of 3 feet around the stove.

- Position barbecue grills at least 10 feet away from siding and deck railings, and out from under eaves and overhanging branches.

Smoking

- Smoke outside, and completely stub out butts in an ashtray or a can filled with sand.

- Soak cigarette butts and ashes in water before throwing them away. Never toss hot cigarette butts or ashes in the trash can.

- Never smoke in a home where oxygen is used, even if it is turned off. Oxygen can be explosive and makes fire burn hotter and faster.

- Be alert—do not smoke in bed. If you are sleepy, have been drinking, or have taken medicine that makes you drowsy, put your cigarette out first.

Electrical and Appliance Safety

- Frayed wires can cause fires. Replace all worn, old, or damaged appliance cords immediately and do not run cords under rugs or furniture.

- If an appliance has a three-prong plug, use it only in a three-slot outlet. Never force it to fit into a two-slot outlet or extension cord.

- Immediately shut off, then professionally replace, light switches that are hot to the touch and lights that flicker.

Portable Space Heaters

- Keep combustible objects at least three feet away from portable heating devices.

- Only buy heaters evaluated by a nationally recognized laboratory, such as Underwriters Laboratories (UL).

- Check to make the portable heater has a thermostat control mechanism and will switch off automatically if the heater falls over.

- Only use crystal clear K-1 kerosene in kerosene heaters. Never overfill it. Use the heater in a well-ventilated room.

Fireplaces and Woodstoves

- Inspect and clean wood stove pipes and chimneys annually, and check monthly for damage or obstructions.

- Use a fireplace screen heavy enough to stop rolling logs and big enough to cover the entire opening of the fireplace to catch flying sparks.

- Make sure the fire is completely out before leaving the house or going to bed.

Children

- Take the mystery out of fire play by teaching children that fire is a tool, not a toy.

- Store matches and lighters out of children's reach and sight, preferably in a locked cabinet.

- Never leave children unattended near operating stoves or burning candles, even for a short time.

More Prevention Tips

- Never use stove range or oven to heat your home.

- Keep combustible and flammable liquids away from heat sources.

- Portable generators should never be used indoors and should only be refueled outdoors or in well-ventilated areas.

Chapter 41

About Fire Extinguishers

It is important to understand that with proper training and education, fire extinguishers can save lives and property. Many of us might not know how or when to use fire extinguishers. You are encouraged to contact your fire department if you would like fire extinguisher training or have any questions. This chapter provides information and tips for using and maintaining fire extinguishers.

Types of Fire Extinguishers

There are five primary types of fire extinguishers, each designed to put out different kinds of fires.

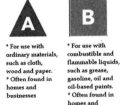

A
* For use with ordinary materials, such as cloth, wood and paper.
* Often found in homes and businesses

B
* For use with combustible and flammable liquids, such as grease, gasoline, oil and oil-based paints.
* Often found in homes and businesses

C
* For use with electrical equipment, such as appliances, tools, or other equipment that is plugged in.
* Often found in homes and businesses

D
* For use with flammable metals
* Often found in factories

K
* For use with vegetable oils, animal oils and fats in cooking appliances.
* Often found in commercial kitchens (restaurants, cafeterias, catering businesses)

Figure 41.1. Five Primary Types of Fire Extinguishers

There are also multipurpose fire extinguishers that might be labeled "B-C" or "A-B-C." Most home improvement stores carry multipurpose fire extinguishers that cover Class A through Class C.

About This Chapter: This chapter includes text excerpted from "Choosing and Using Fire Extinguishers," U.S. Fire Administration (FA), December 12, 2017.

When to Use a Fire Extinguisher

Fire extinguishers can be helpful on a small fire. Find below a checklist that will help you to prepare to use a fire extinguisher on a potential fire.

- Have I alerted others in the building that there is a fire?

- Has someone called the fire department?

- Am I physically able to use a fire extinguisher?

- Is the fire small and contained in a single object (such as a pan or a wastebasket)?

- Am I safe from the fire's toxic smoke?

- Do I have a clear escape route?

Use a fire extinguisher when all of these questions are answered "yes." If you are unsure about whether or not it is safe to use a fire extinguisher, and for all other situations, alert others, leave the building, and call 911 from a mobile or neighbor's phone. However, children are not recommended to use fire extinguishers.

How to Use a Fire Extinguisher

When operating a fire extinguisher, you should remember the word PASS:

- **Pull the pin.** Hold the extinguisher with the nozzle pointing away from you and release the locking mechanism.

- **Aim low.** Point the extinguisher at the base of the fire.

- **Squeeze** the lever slowly and evenly.

- **Sweep** the nozzle from side-to-side.

The Importance of Fire Extinguisher Maintenance

You should check fire extinguishers for:

- **Easy access in an emergency.** Be sure nothing is blocking or limiting your ability to reach it.

- **The recommended pressure levels.** Many extinguishers have gauges that show when pressure is too high or too low.

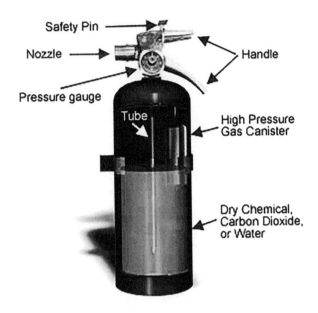

Figure 41.2. Portable Fire Extinguisher *(Source: "Emergency Standards—Portable Fire Extinguishers," Occupational Safety and Health Administration (OSHA).)*

- **Working parts.** Make sure the can, hoses and nozzles aren't damaged, dented, or rusted.

- **Cleanliness.** Remove any dust, oil, or grease that might be on the outside of the extinguisher.

- **Guidelines and instructions.** Some extinguishers need to be shaken monthly; others need to be pressure tested every few years.

Chapter 42

The Dangers of Carbon Monoxide

Carbon monoxide (CO) is the "invisible" killer. It is a colorless and odorless gas. Every year more than 100 people in the United States die from unintentional exposure to carbon monoxide associated with consumer products.

What Is Carbon Monoxide?

Carbon monoxide is produced by burning fuel. Therefore, any fuel-burning appliance in your home is a potential CO source.

When cooking or heating appliances are kept in good working order, they produce little CO. Improperly operating appliances can produce fatal CO concentrations in your home.

Running a car or generator in an attached garage can cause fatal CO poisoning in the home, as can running a generator or burning charcoal in the basement, crawlspace, or living area of the home.

Who Is at Risk from Carbon Monoxide Poisoning?

Everyone is at risk for carbon monoxide (CO) poisoning. Infants, the elderly, people with chronic heart disease, anemia, or breathing problems are more likely to get sick from CO. Each year, more than 400 Americans die from unintentional CO poisoning not linked to fires, more than 20,000 visit the emergency room, and more than 4,000 are hospitalized.

(Source: "Carbon Monoxide Poisoning—Frequently Asked Questions," Centers for Disease Control and Prevention (CDC).)

About This Chapter: This chapter includes text excerpted from "The "Invisible" Killer," U.S. Consumer Product Safety Commission (CPSC), September 25, 2016.

Sources of and Clues to a Possible Carbon Monoxide Problem

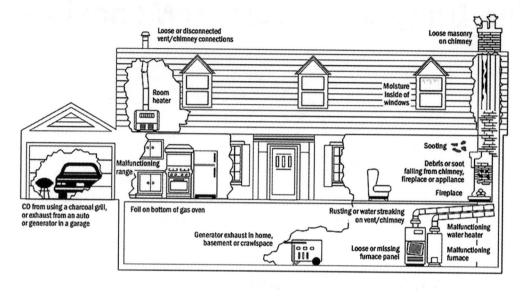

Figure 42.1. Possible Sources of Carbon Monoxide

Carbon Monoxide Clues You Can See

- Rusting or water streaking on vent/chimney

- Loose or missing furnace panel

- Sooting

- Debris or soot falling from chimney, fireplace, or appliances

- Loose or disconnected vent/chimney, fireplace, or appliance

- Loose masonry on chimney

- Moisture inside of windows

Carbon Monoxide Clues You Cannot See

- Internal appliance damage or malfunctioning components

- Improper burner adjustments

- Hidden blockage or damage in chimneys

234

Only a trained service technician can detect hidden problems and correct these conditions.

- Carbon monoxide poisoning symptoms have been experienced when you are home, but they lessen or disappear when you are away from home.

Warnings

- Never leave a car running in a garage, even with the garage door open.

- Never run a generator in the home, garage, or crawlspace. Opening doors and windows or using fans will not prevent CO buildup in the home. When running a generator out-doors, keep it away from open windows and doors.

- Never burn charcoal in homes, tents, vehicles, or garages.

- Never install or service combustion appliances without proper knowledge, skills, and tools.

- Never use a gas range, oven, or dryer for heating.

- Never put foil on the bottom of a gas oven because it interferes with combustion.

- Never operate an unvented gas-burning appliance in a closed room or in a room in which you are sleeping.

Symptoms of Carbon Monoxide Poisoning

The initial symptoms of CO poisoning are similar to the flu (but without the fever). They include:

- Headache

- Fatigue

- Shortness of breath

- Nausea

- Dizziness

If you suspect that you are experiencing CO poisoning, get fresh air immediately. Leave the home, and call for assistance from a neighbor's home. You could lose consciousness and die from CO poisoning if you stay in the home.

Get medical attention immediately, and inform the medical staff that CO poisoning is suspected. Call the fire department to determine when it is safe to reenter the home.

What Should You Do?

Proper installation, operation, and maintenance of fuel-burning appliances in the home is the most important factor in reducing the risk of CO poisoning. Make sure appliances are installed according to the manufacturer's instructions and the local codes. Most appliances should be installed by professionals. Always follow the appliance manufacturer's directions for safe operation.

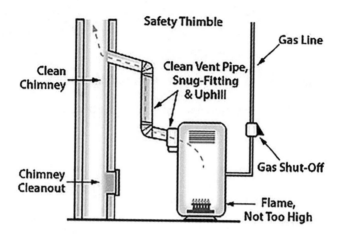

Figure 42.2. Safe Way to Connect Heating Equipment to the Chimney *(Source: "Carbon Monoxide Poisoning—Frequently Asked Questions," Centers for Disease Control and Prevention (CDC).)*

Have the heating system (including chimneys and vents) inspected and serviced annually by a trained service technician. Examine vents and chimneys regularly for improper connections, visible cracks, rust, or stains.

Look for problems that could indicate improper appliance operation:

• Decreased hot water supply

• Furnace unable to heat the house or runs continuously

• Sooting, especially on appliances and vents

• An unfamiliar or burning odor

• Increased moisture inside of windows

Operate portable generators outdoors and away from open doors, windows, and vents that could allow CO to come indoors.

In addition, install battery-operated CO alarms or plug-in CO alarms with battery backup in your home. Every home should have a CO alarm in the hallway near the bedrooms in each separate sleeping area. The CO alarms should be certified to the requirements of the most recent Underwriters Laboratories (UL), International Accounting Standards (IAS), or Canadian Standards Association (CSA) standard for CO alarms. Test your CO alarms frequently, and replace dead batteries. A CO alarm can provide added protection but is no substitute for proper installation, use, and upkeep of appliances that are potential CO sources.

Chapter 43

Poison Prevention Tips

Poisons are all around us and can affect anyone, anywhere, at any time of life. Protect yourself and others from being poisoned by learning what a poison is, who is at risk, and how to prevent a poisoning from happening.

What Is a Poison?

A poison is anything that can harm someone if it is:

- Used in the wrong way

- Used by the wrong person

- Used in the wrong amount

Some poisons may be harmful if they come into direct contact with your eyes or skin. Others may be toxic if you breathe them or swallow them.

Poisons can come in four forms:

- **Solids,** such as pain medicine pills or tablets

- **Liquids,** such as household cleaners, including bleach

- **Sprays,** such as spray cleaners

- **Gases,** such as carbon monoxide, or CO

About This Chapter: This chapter includes text excerpted from "Poison Info—Poison Help," Health Resources and Services Administration (HRSA), August 10, 2010. Reviewed July 2019.

Most consumer products are safe if label directions are followed, but some can be poisonous if used incorrectly.

Who Is at Risk for Poisoning?

You may think that poisoning affects only a certain group of people, such as young children or older adults. This, however, is not true. Anyone, regardless of their age, race, ethnicity, or career, can be poisoned. Poisonings happen more often than you think.

In 2008, 2.5 million people approached a poison center because someone had been exposed to a poison. Children under 6 years of age accounted for half of all human poison exposures reported to poison centers. However, adults are also at risk. That year, more than three-quarters of all poisoning deaths reported to poison centers occurred among people between 20 and 59 years of age.

What Are the Risks throughout Life?

Certain kinds of poisonings are common among specific age groups. For example, older adults specifically need to be aware of the poisoning risks involved with taking prescription medications. Children are commonly poisoned through painkillers, cosmetics, personal care or cleaning products, pest killers, and plants. Preteens through older adults are commonly poisoned through herbal products, prescription drugs, alcohol, over-the-counter (OTC) medicines, and spoiled food.

People of all ages may be stung by a bee, splashed with a chemical, or exposed to CO in their homes. People also may use a cleaning product without gloves.

What You Can Do

If someone may have been poisoned, call the toll-free Poison Helpline (800-222-1222), which connects you to your local poison center, to speak with a poison expert right away. This expert can give you advice on first aid and may save you from a visit to the emergency room.

Below is a checklist to help you in the event of a poisoning:

First Steps

- If the person is not breathing, call 911.

- If the person inhaled poison, get her or him fresh air right away.

- If the person has poison on the skin, take off any clothing the poison touched. Rinse skin with running water for 15 to 20 minutes.

- If the person has poison in the eyes, rinse their eyes with running water for 15 to 20 minutes.

- Do not use activated charcoal when you think someone may have been poisoned.

Calling the Poison Helpline

- Do not wait for signs of poisoning before calling the Poison Helpline.

- Stay calm. Not all medicines, chemicals, or household products are poisonous. Not all contact with poison results in poisoning.

- Make sure to have the container of the product you think caused the poisoning nearby. The label has important information.

Be Ready to Tell the Expert on the Phone

- The exposed person's age and weight

- Known health conditions or problems

- The product involved

- How the product contacted the person (for example, by mouth, by inhaling, through the skin, or through the eyes)

- How long ago the poison contacted the person

- What first aid has already been given

- Whether the person has vomited

- Your exact location and how long it would take you to get to a hospital

Help Prevent Poisonings

- Learn how to poison proof your home and reduce the risk of poisoning.

- Talk about poisons so others know what to do too.

- Prevent pill abuse and theft by ridding your home of potentially dangerous expired, unused, and unwanted prescription drugs.

Winter Tips

The following tips are primarily for the Winter season, but be aware of them year round.

Many people think poinsettias and Christmas cacti are poisonous. They are not, but mistletoe should be kept where it cannot be reached by young children or pets. Here are some other dangers to watch out for in Winter.

Antifreeze

- Antifreeze is a poisonous liquid used in cars. It has a sweet taste that children and animals like. If even a little is swallowed, it can be harmful and can cause kidney damage and death.

- Keep antifreeze, household cleaners, and all chemicals in the containers they came in with a tight cap, and keep them away from children and pets.

- Before throwing away an antifreeze container, rinse it with water, and replace the safety cap.

Snow Salt

- Salt used on driveways and sidewalks in the Winter can harm a pet or child if eaten.
- Store such salt out of reach and in a locked cabinet.

Mercury

- Avoid using glass mercury thermometers. They can break in a child's mouth. Instead, use a digital thermometer.
- Stay with children when taking their temperature.
- Spilled mercury should be cleaned up properly as it is a hazardous waste. Call the Poison Helpline or your local health department for advice.

Carbon Monoxide

Carbon monoxide is a poisonous gas and has no color, odor, or taste. All fuel-burning devices make CO, mostly when they are not working properly or are not used in a ventilated space. CO can collect in closed areas. Sources of CO include gas furnaces, gas water heaters, gas stoves, gas ovens, kerosene space heaters, wood and gas fireplaces, wood-burning stoves, power generators, and car engines.

People at the greatest risk for CO poisoning include pregnant women, infants, young children, older people, people with diseases that affect breathing, and people with heart disease.

Signs of CO poisoning are similar to signs of the flu and some cold-weather viruses: headaches, nausea, vomiting, dizziness, and confusion.

To prevent CO poisoning in your home:

- Have at least one CO detector in your home. The best places for a CO detector are near bedrooms and close to furnaces.

- Have your heating system, vents, and chimney checked every year by experts.

- Always follow product instructions for installing and repairing appliances that burn fuel.

- Never burn charcoal inside a house or garage.

- Never use a gas oven to heat a house or apartment or use unvented fuel-burning devices indoors.

- Never run a car in a closed garage.

Spring Tips

The following tips are primarily for the Spring season, but be aware of them all year. As you begin Spring cleaning and work on the yard, follow these simple tips to keep your family safe.

Household Cleaners and Other Products

- Keep household cleaners and potentially poisonous substances in the containers they came in.

- Do not use food containers (such as cups or bottles) to store household cleaners and other chemicals or products.

- Store strong chemicals away from food. Many poisonings occur when one product is mistaken for another.

- Read and follow the directions for use of the products and their disposal. Do this before using the products. Follow the advice carefully.

- Never mix chemicals or household cleaners or detergents. Doing so can create a poisonous gas.

- Turn on fans and open windows when using chemicals or household cleaners.

- Never sniff containers to see what is inside.

- When spraying chemicals, direct the spray nozzle away from people and pets.

- Discard old or outdated products. First aid advice on containers may be incorrect and outdated.

- Call the Poison Helpline to double check first aid information.

- Even in small amounts, windshield wiper fluid is poisonous. If swallowed, it can cause blindness or death to people and pets. Use it carefully to avoid spraying it in someone's face.

- Chemicals can burn the skin. Drain openers, toilet cleaners, rust removers, and oven cleaners can cause such burns.

- Liquids made from petroleum, such as gasoline, kerosene, charcoal lighter fluid, paint thinner, baby oil, lamp oil, and furniture polish, are poisonous.

- If these items are swallowed, they can easily get into the lungs. Even a small amount can cause breathing problems. The liquid coats the inside of the lungs and prevents oxygen from entering the bloodstream.

- Tell children that they should ask a grown-up if they are not sure if something is dangerous. Tell them to stay away from things used to clean the house, clothes, or car.

Pesticides

- Pesticides (pest killers) can be taken in through the skin or inhaled and can be extremely poisonous. Even leather shoes and gloves do not offer full protection.

- Stay away from areas that have been sprayed until the spray has dried or for at least one hour.

- Wear protective clothing when using bug spray or other spray products. Put on a long-sleeve shirt, long pants, socks, shoes, and gloves. Remove and wash clothing after using chemicals.

- If pesticides are splashed onto the skin, rinse with running water for 15 to 20 minutes. If pesticide contacts clothing, take off the clothing before rinsing skin.

- Many garden chemicals are poisonous if swallowed or inhaled by children and adults.

Mushrooms

- Only experts can tell poisonous mushrooms from safe mushrooms.

- Poisonous mushrooms, called "death caps," often grow in yards and parks.

- Eating even a few bites of certain mushrooms can cause liver damage that can kill you.

Summer Tips

The following tips are primarily for the Summer season, but be aware of them year round.

Summer is a time for enjoying the outdoors. However, it is important to remember that these favored months can bring an increase in the incidence of poisoning accidents.

Food Poisoning

- Always wash hands and counters before preparing food. Use clean utensils for cooking and serving.

- Store, cook, and reheat food at the proper temperatures.

- Refrigerated foods should not be left out at temperatures above 40°F (5°C). The following foods, and others, can quickly spoil and become unsafe: party platters, meat, poultry, seafood, dairy products, eggs, mayonnaise, and cooked vegetables.

- Do not let food sit out at room temperature for more than two hours.

- Wash hands, cutting boards, utensils, and dishes with hot, soapy water after handling raw meat, poultry, or seafood.

- Watch for signs of food poisoning. They include fever, headache, diarrhea, stomach pains, nausea, and vomiting.

Mushrooms

- Only experts can tell poisonous mushrooms from safe mushrooms.

- Poisonous mushrooms, called "death caps," often grow in yards and parks.

- Eating even a few bites of certain mushrooms can cause liver damage that can kill you.

Plants

- If you are allergic to poison ivy, poison oak, or poison sumac, touching it can cause blisters on your skin.

- Be sure that everyone in your family can identify these plants. Remember the phrase, " leaves of three, let it be."

- If someone touches one of these plants, rinse the skin right away with running water for at least five minutes.

- Unless you are a plant expert, do not pick your own foods to eat in the wild.

- Poison center experts may not be able to identify plants on the phone, so it is important before poisoning occurs to learn the names of plants around your home.

Insect Bites

- Be alert to insects that may bite or sting, particularly bees, wasps, hornets, and yellow jackets. After a sting, the skin will show redness and swelling, and it may be itchy and painful.

- Insect stings may cause serious problems and even death for those who are allergic to them.

- Go to a hospital right away if you are stung and have any of these signs: hives, dizziness, breathing trouble, or swelling around eyes and mouth.

Snakebites

- If a poisonous snake bites you or someone you know, call the Poison Helpline right away.

- The experts at your poison center will determine if the snake is poisonous. They will tell you what signs to watch for and what to do.

- If the snake is not poisonous, you will need to wash the wound. Check with your doctor to find out if you need a tetanus booster shot.

Spider Bites

- Most spider and tick bites do not cause harm, but there are some spiders that can cause illness in some people. Two common spiders that can harm you are the female black widow and the brown recluse. A bite from one of these spiders can cause serious problems in a child, an older adult, or a person in poor health, but it rarely causes death.

- The female black widow is a black, shiny spider. It has a red or orange hourglass shape on its underside. Within two hours after being bitten by one, you may feel stomach pain, dizziness, and muscle stiffness. You may have trouble breathing.

- The brown recluse is a yellowish-tan to dark brown spider. It has a small body and long legs. The brown recluse has a dark violin shape on its body. Within 36 hours after being bitten, you may see or feel signs of poisoning. You may feel restless and have fever, chills, nausea, weakness, a rash, or joint pain. A blister or wound may develop at the bite site, possibly in the shape of a bull's eye (a blister with rings around). If the wound worsens, see a doctor. Most likely you will not need antibiotics.

- States known to be home to the brown recluse are Alabama, Arkansas, Florida, Georgia, Iowa, Illinois, Indiana, Kansas, Kentucky, Louisiana, Missouri, Mississippi, North Carolina, Nebraska, New Mexico, Ohio, Oklahoma, South Carolina, Tennessee, and Texas.

Insect Spray or Lotion

Be sure to check the label on any insect repellent. Be aware that most contain N,N-diethyl-meta-toluamide (DEET), which can be dangerous in large quantities.

- Use separate products when there is a need for insect spray and sunscreen.

- Follow the label instructions.

- Do not use sunscreen that contains DEET.

- Repeatedly applying a product with DEET can increase the risk of harmful effects.

- For most products, after returning indoors, wash treated skin with soap and water.

- Check the label of the product you are using for more advice.

Alcoholic Drinks and Products

- Alcohol can be a deadly poison for children because they are small, and their livers are not fully developed. All of the following are dangerous for children: beer, wine, mixed drinks, other alcoholic beverages, facial cleaners, and mouthwash. Therefore, do not leave products containing alcohol where children can reach them.

- Alcohol will make a child sleepy. The child can develop low blood sugar. This can lead to seizures, coma, and death.

- Be alert at parties and gatherings. Children may find cups containing leftover alcohol within their reach.

Other Poison Risks to Watch For

- Lighter fluid, gasoline, torch and lamp oils can be deadly if swallowed. Watch children closely at all times when these are being used.

- Use camp stoves, grills, and generators outside, never inside buildings or tents.

- Inhaling chlorine products can irritate the respiratory system. Homeowners who have swimming pools should store pool chemicals in a safe and secure place, out of children's reach.

Fall Tips

The following tips are primarily for the Fall season, but be aware of them all year.

Kids are back in school. Cold and flu season is here. Holidays are just around the corner—be mindful of food safety concerns surrounding your family. Here are some other tips to help you prevent poisonings during this busy time of year.

Medicines

- Keep medicines, vitamins, diet supplements, and household products in the containers they came in (i.e., tight, possibly child-proof lids).

- Keep them locked up where children cannot see or reach them, particularly those medicines that taste, smell, or look like candy or drinks. Do this at home and when traveling.

- Tell your doctor about all the medicines you are taking and be careful when taking multiple prescriptions.

- Be sure you are not using two or more products that contain the same drug.

- It is common to overdose on the drug acetaminophen, so be extra careful.

- Read and follow the directions and warnings on all labels before taking medicine.

- If you have questions about how to use your medicine, call your doctor or pharmacist or call the Poison Helpline.

- Talk to your doctor before taking any food supplements (such as vitamins, minerals, or herbs).

- Never take medicine in the dark.

- Never take other people's prescription drugs. Take only those that are prescribed for you.

- Products, such as medicine, that taste, smell, or look like candy or drinks may attract children. Be sure to keep these products out of sight. Keep them out of reach and locked up.

- Children learn by imitating adults. Children who see adults taking medicine will try to do the same thing.

- Do you have the medicine you no longer need or that has expired? Get rid of medicines that have expired or are no longer needed. Ask your local pharmacist how you can return unused, unneeded, or expired prescription drugs to pharmaceutical take-back locations for safe disposal. If this is not available, take the unused, unneeded, or expired prescription drugs out of their original containers. Mix the drugs with an undesirable substance, such as kitty litter, and put them in waterproof containers, such as empty cans or sealable bags, to make sure that they are not found and used by people or animals. Throw these containers in the trash. Your poison center may have updated advice for your area, call 800-222-1222. The Drug Enforcement Administration (DEA) and its national and community partners hold their National Prescription Take-Back Day in late April and October.

Mushrooms

- Only experts can tell poisonous mushrooms from safe mushrooms.

- Eating even a few bites of certain mushrooms can cause liver damage that can kill you.

- Poisonous mushrooms, called "death caps," often grow in yards and parks.

Berries

- Berries may attract children. Some berries that can harm people do not harm birds and other animals.

- If you think someone ate berries from a plant, right away call the Poison Helpline (800-222-1222), which connects you to your local poison center. Poison center experts probably will not be able to identify the plant on the phone.

- A greenhouse or plant nursery can help identify your plants, so learn the names of the plants around your home just in case.

- Back to school and art supplies

- Children often use art products (e.g., glue, paint, ink) at home, school, and day care. These art products are mixtures of chemicals. They can be dangerous if not used correctly, stored properly, or expired.

- Make sure children use art products safely by reading labels carefully, following the directions for safe use and disposal, and cleaning up tables, desks, and counters appropriately.

- Young children are likely to put pretty, colorful art products in their mouths. Additionally, if a product is splashed into the eyes or spilled onto skin, right away call the Poison Helpline (800-222-1222), which connects you to your local poison center.

- Do not eat or drink while using art products.

- Never use products for painting skin unless the product says it is safe to do so.

- Never use products to decorate food unless the product says it is safe to do so.

- Keep art products in the containers they came in.

Carbon Monoxide

- Fall is usually the time we turn on heaters and generators. Make sure your heating system is running smoothly and the carbon monoxide detector has fresh batteries.

Chapter 44

Electrical and Power Outage Safety

Whenever you work with power tools or on electrical circuits, there is a risk of electrical hazards, especially electrical shock. Anyone can be exposed to these hazards at home or at work. Coming in contact with an electrical voltage can cause current to flow through the body, resulting in electrical shock and burns. Serious injury or even death may occur. As a source of energy, electricity is used without much thought about the hazards it can cause. Because electricity is a familiar part of our lives, it often is not treated with enough caution.

According to the U.S. Bureau of Labor Statistics' (BLS) Census of Fatal Occupational Injuries Research File for 1992 to 2005, electrocution is the 5th leading cause of work-related deaths for 16- to 19-year-olds, after motor vehicle deaths, contact with objects and equipment, workplace homicide, and falls. Electrocution is the cause of 7 percent of all workplace deaths among young workers aged 16 to 19, causing an average of 10 deaths per year.

How Is an Electrical Shock Received?

An electrical shock is received when electrical current passes through the body. Current will pass through the body in a variety of situations. Whenever two wires are at different voltages, current will pass between them if they are connected. Your body can connect the wires if you touch both of them at the same time. Current will pass through your body.

About This Chapter: Text in this chapter begins with excerpts from "Electrical Safety: Safety and Health for Electrical Trades," Centers for Disease Control and Prevention (CDC), April 1, 2009. Reviewed July 2019; Text beginning with the heading "Power Outrages" is excerpted from "What You Need to Know When the Power Goes Out Unexpectedly," Centers for Disease Control and Prevention (CDC), October 17, 2017.

In most household wiring, the black wires and the red wires are at 120 volts. The white wires are at 0 volts because they are connected to ground. The connection to ground is often through a conducting ground rod driven into the earth. The connection can also be made through a buried metal water pipe. If you come in contact with an energized black wire—and you are also in contact with the neutral white wire—current will pass through your body. You will receive an electrical shock.

If you are in contact with a live wire or any live component of an energized electrical device—and also in contact with any grounded object—you will receive a shock. Plumbing is often grounded. Metal electrical boxes and conduit are grounded.

Your risk of receiving a shock is greater if you stand in a puddle of water. But, you do not even have to be standing in water to be at risk. Wet clothing, high humidity, and perspiration also increase your chances of being electrocuted. Of course, there is always a chance of electrocution, even in dry conditions.

You can even receive a shock when you are not in contact with an electrical ground. Contact with both live wires of a 240-volt cable will deliver a shock. (This type of shock can occur because one live wire may be at +120 volts while the other is at -120 volts during an alternating current cycle—a difference of 240 volts.). You can also receive a shock from electrical components that are not grounded properly. Even contact with another person who is receiving an electrical shock may cause you to be shocked.

Dangers of Electrical Shock

The severity of injury from electrical shock depends on the amount of electrical current and the length of time the current passes through the body. For example, 1/10 of an ampere (amp) of electricity going through the body for just 2 seconds is enough to cause death. The amount of internal current a person can withstand and still be able to control the muscles of the arm and hand can be less than 10 milliamperes (milliamps or mA). Currents above 10 mA can paralyze or "freeze" muscles. When this "freezing" happens, a person is no longer able to release a tool, wire, or other object. In fact, the electrified object may be held even more tightly, resulting in longer exposure to the shocking current. For this reason, hand-held tools that give a shock can be very dangerous. If you can't let go of the tool, current continues through your body for a longer time, which can lead to respiratory paralysis (the muscles that control breathing cannot move). You stop breathing for a period of time. People have stopped breathing when shocked with currents from voltages as low as 49 volts. Usually, it takes about 30 mA of current to cause respiratory paralysis.

Currents greater than 75 mA cause ventricular fibrillation (very rapid, ineffective heart-beat). This condition will cause death within a few minutes unless a special device called a "defibrillator" is used to save the victim. Heart paralysis occurs at 4 amps, which means the heart does not pump at all. Tissue is burned with currents greater than 5 amps. Longer exposure times increase the danger to the shock victim. For example, a current of 100 mA applied for 3 seconds is as dangerous as a current of 900 mA applied for a fraction of a second (0.03 seconds). The muscle structure of the person also makes a difference. People with less muscle tissue are typically affected at lower current levels. Even low voltages can be extremely dangerous because the degree of injury depends not only on the amount of current but also on the length of time the body is in contact with the circuit.

Sometimes high voltages lead to additional injuries. High voltages can cause violent muscular contractions. You may lose your balance and fall, which can cause injury or even death if you fall into machinery that can crush you. High voltages can also cause severe burns.

At 600 volts, the current through the body may be as great as 4 amps, causing damage to internal organs such as the heart. High voltages also produce burns. In addition, internal blood vessels may clot. Nerves in the area of the contact point may be damaged. Muscle contractions may cause bone fractures from either the contractions themselves or from falls.

A severe shock can cause much more damage to the body than is visible. A person may suffer internal bleeding and destruction of tissues, nerves, and muscles. Sometimes the hidden injuries caused by electrical shock result in a delayed death. Shock is often only the beginning of a chain of events. Even if the electrical current is too small to cause injury, your reaction to the shock may cause you to fall, resulting in bruises, broken bones, or even death.

The length of time of the shock greatly affects the amount of injury. If the shock is short in duration, it may only be painful. A longer shock (lasting a few seconds) could be fatal if the level of current is high enough to cause the heart to go into ventricular fibrillation. This is not much current when you realize that a small power drill uses 30 times as much current as what will kill. At relatively high currents, death is certain if the shock is long enough. However, if the shock is short and the heart has not been damaged, a normal heartbeat may resume if contact with the electrical current is eliminated. (This type of recovery is rare.)

The amount of current passing through the body also affects the severity of an electrical shock. Greater voltages produce greater currents. So, there is greater danger from higher voltages. Resistance hinders current. The lower the resistance (or impedance in AC circuits), the greater the current flow will be. Dry skin may have a resistance of 100,000 ohms or more. Wet skin may have a resistance of only 1,000 ohms. Wet working conditions or broken skin will drastically reduce resistance. The low resistance of wet skin allows current to pass into the body more easily and give a greater shock. When more force is applied to the contact point or when the contact area is larger, the resistance is lower, causing stronger shocks.

The path of the electrical current through the body affects the severity of the shock. Currents through the heart or nervous system are most dangerous. If you contact a live wire with your head, your nervous system may be damaged. Contacting a live electrical part with one hand—while you are grounded at the other side of your body—will cause electrical current to pass across your chest, possibly injuring your heart and lungs.

There have been cases where an arm or leg is severely burned by high-voltage electrical current to the point of coming off, and the victim is not electrocuted. In these cases, the current passes through only a part of the limb before it goes out of the body and into another conductor. Therefore, the current does not go through the chest area and may not cause death, even though the victim is severely disfigured. If the current does go through the chest, the person will almost surely be electrocuted. A large number of serious electrical injuries involve current passing from the hands to the feet. Such a path involves both the heart and lungs. This type of shock is often fatal.

Burns Caused by Electricity

The most common shock-related, nonfatal injury is a burn. Burns caused by electricity may be of three types: electrical burns, arc burns, and thermal contact burns. Electrical burns can result when a person touches electrical wiring or equipment that is used or maintained improperly. Typically, such burns occur on the hands. Electrical burns are one of the most serious injuries you can receive. They need to be given immediate attention. Additionally, clothing may catch fire and a thermal burn may result from the heat of the fire.

Arc Blasts

Arc-blasts occur when powerful, high-amperage currents arc through the air. Arcing is the luminous electrical discharge that occurs when high voltages exist across a gap between conductors and current travels through the air. This situation is often caused by equipment failure due to abuse or fatigue. Temperatures as high as 35,000 °F have been reached in arc-blasts. A common example of arcing is the flash you sometimes see when you turn a light switch on or off. This is not dangerous because of the low voltage.

There are three primary hazards associated with an arc-blast.

- Arcing gives off thermal radiation (heat) and intense light, which can cause burns. Several factors affect the degree of injury, including skin color, area of skin exposed, and type of clothing worn. Proper clothing, work distances, and over-current protection can reduce the risk of such a burn.

- A high-voltage arc can produce a considerable pressure wave blast. A person 2 feet away from a 25,000-amp arc feels a force of about 480 pounds on the front of the body. In addition, such an explosion can cause serious ear damage and memory loss due to concussion. Sometimes the pressure wave throws the victim away from the arc-blast. While this may reduce further exposure to the thermal energy, serious physical injury may result. The pressure wave can propel large objects over great distances. In some cases, the pressure wave has enough force to snap off the heads of steel bolts and knock over walls.

- A high-voltage arc can also cause many of the copper and aluminum components in electrical equipment to melt. These droplets of molten metal can be blasted great distances by the pressure wave. Although these droplets harden rapidly, they can still be hot enough to cause serious burns or cause ordinary clothing to catch fire, even if you are 10 feet or more away.

Thermal burns may result if an explosion occurs when electricity ignites an explosive mixture of material in the air. This ignition can result from the buildup of combustible vapors, gases, or dusts. Occupational Safety and Health Administration (OSHA) standards, National Fire Protection Association (NFPA) standards, and other safety standards give precise safety requirements for the operation of electrical systems and equipment in such dangerous areas. Ignition can also be caused by overheated conductors or equipment, or by normal arcing at switch contacts or in circuit breakers.

Electrical Fires

Electricity is one of the most common causes of fires and thermal burns in homes and workplaces. Defective or misused electrical equipment is a major cause of electrical fires. If there is a small electrical fire, be sure to use only a Class C or multipurpose (ABC) fire extinguisher, or you might make the problem worse. All fire extinguishers are marked with letter(s) that tell you the kinds of fires they can put out. Some extinguishers contain symbols, too.

The letters and symbols are explained in the figure 44.1 (including suggestions on how to remember them).

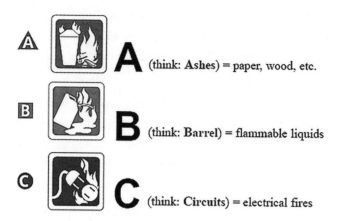

(think: Ashes) = paper, wood, etc.

(think: Barrel) = flammable liquids

(think: Circuits) = electrical fires

Figure 44.1. Symbols on Fire Extinguisher

First Aid for Electric Shock

Shut off the electrical current if the victim is still in contact with the energized circuit. While you do this, have someone else call for help. If you cannot get to the switchgear quickly, pry the victim from the circuit with something that does not conduct electricity such as dry wood. Do not touch the victim yourself if she or he is still in contact with an electrical circuit! You do not want to be a victim, too!

Do not leave the victim unless there is absolutely no other option. You should stay with the victim while emergency medical services (EMS) are contacted. The caller should come back to you afterward to verify that the call was made. If the victim is not breathing, does not have a heartbeat, or is badly injured, quick response by a team of emergency medical technicians (EMTs) or paramedics gives the best chance for survival.

Once you know that electrical current is no longer flowing through the victim, call out to the victim to see if she or he is conscious (awake). If the victim is conscious, tell the victim not to move. It is possible for a shock victim to be seriously injured but not realize it. Quickly examine the victim for signs of major bleeding. If there is a lot of bleeding, place a cloth (such as a handkerchief or bandanna) over the wound and apply pressure. If the wound is in an arm or leg and keeps bleeding a lot, gently elevate the injured area while keeping pressure on the wound. Keep the victim warm and talk to her or him until help arrives.

If the victim is unconscious, check for signs of breathing. While you do this, move the victim as little as possible. If the victim is not breathing, someone trained in CPR should begin artificial breathing, then check to see if the victim has a pulse. Quick action is essential! To be effective, CPR must be performed within 4 minutes of the shock.

You also need to know the location of:

- Electricity shut-offs ("kill switches")

- First-aid supplies

- A telephone so you can find them quickly in an emergency

Power Outrages

This chapter also offers tips to help you prepare for and cope with sudden loss of power.

Food Safety

If the power is out for less than four hours, then the food in your refrigerator and freezer will be safe to consume. While the power is out, keep the refrigerator and freezer doors closed as much as possible to keep food cold for longer.

Safe Drinking Water

When the power goes out, water purification systems may not be functioning fully. Safe water for drinking, cooking, and personal hygiene includes bottled, boiled, or treated water. Your state, local, or tribal health department can make specific recommendations for boiling or treating water in your area.

Medications

Some drugs require refrigeration to keep their strength, including many liquid drugs.

- When the power is out for a day or more, throw away any medication that should be refrigerated, unless the drug's label says otherwise.

- If a life depends on the refrigerated drugs, but the medications have been at room temperature, use them only until a new supply is available.

- Replace all refrigerated drugs as soon as possible.

Extreme Heat

Be aware of yours and others' risk for heat stroke, heat exhaustion, heat cramps, and fainting.

Heat stroke is the most serious heat illness. It happens when the body cannot control its own temperature, and its temperature rises rapidly. Sweating fails, and the body cannot cool down. Body temperature may rise to 106°F or higher within 10 to 15 minutes. Heat stroke can cause death or permanent disability if emergency care is not given.

If air conditioning is not available in your home:

- Contact your local health department or locate an air-conditioned shelter in your area.

- Spend some time at a shopping mall or public library—even a few hours spent in air conditioning can help.

- Take cool showers or baths.

- Do not rely solely on fans to keep you cool. While electric fans might provide some comfort, when temperatures are really hot, they would not prevent heat-related illness.

Extreme Cold

- Hypothermia happens when a person's core body temperature is lower than 35°C (95°F).

Power Line Hazards and Cars

If a power line falls on a car, you should stay inside the vehicle. This is the safest place to stay. Warn people not to touch the car or the line. Call or ask someone to call the local utility company and emergency services.

The only circumstance in which you should consider leaving a car that is in contact with a downed power line is if the vehicle catches on fire. Open the door. Do not step out of the car. You may receive a shock. Instead, jump free of the car so that your body clears the vehicle before touching the ground. Once you clear the car, shuffle at least 50 feet away, with both feet on the ground.

As in all power-line-related emergencies, call for help immediately by dialing 911 or call your electric utility company's service center/dispatch office.

Do not try to help someone else from the car while you are standing on the ground.

Dangers of Gasoline Siphoning

Gasoline may be in short supply before, during, and after natural disasters, such as hurricanes and floods. When there is not enough gasoline, people may want to take gasoline from one container and put it into another. This can be done by siphoning.

- Siphoning gasoline can harm your health. Do not try to siphon gasoline. It can cause serious injury or illness

- Siphoning is when you use your mouth or a pump to suck a liquid such as gasoline out of one container, such as a gas tank, through a funnel or tube and into another container.

- Possible injuries and illness from any form of siphoning include:

  - Burns and injury from unintentional combustion of gasoline and/or gasoline vapors. This may happen if the gasoline or its vapors come into contact with a lit cigarette or static electricity.

  - Confusion, drowsiness, headache, or problems concentrating from breathing gasoline vapors

  - Irritation of skin, eye, or mucous membranes on contact

- Other possible injuries and illness from siphoning when you use your mouth for suction include:

  - Lung damage, if gasoline is inhaled into the lungs (aspiration) during mouth-based siphoning

  - Gastrointestinal (GI) signs and symptoms, such as nausea, vomiting, and stomach pain, if any gasoline is swallowed

  - Irritation of mucous membranes inside your mouth, throat, and stomach on contact

- If you do breathe gasoline fumes or swallow gasoline and feel ill, see a doctor and/or call the poison center for help at 800-222-1222.

Be Prepared for an Emergency

The Centers for Disease Control and Prevention (CDC) recommends that people make an emergency plan that includes a disaster supply kit. This kit should include enough water, dried and canned food, and emergency supplies (flashlights, batteries, first-aid supplies, prescription medicines, and a digital thermometer) to last at least three days. Use battery-powered flashlights and lanterns rather than candles, gas lanterns, or torches (to minimize the risk of fire).

Emergency Supplies List

- ☐ 3-day supply of non-perishable food (dried fruit, canned tuna fish, peanut butter, etc.)
- ☐ Can opener
- ☐ First aid kit
- ☐ Sleeping bag or warm blanket for everyone in your family
- ☐ Change of clothes to last 3 days, including sturdy shoes; consider the weather where you live
- ☐ Matches in a waterproof container (let a grown up handle these)
- ☐ Toothbrush, toothpaste, soap
- ☐ Paper plates, plastic cups and utensils, paper towels

- ☐ Water – at least a gallon per person, per day
- ☐ Battery-powered or hand-cranked radio with extra batteries
- ☐ Flashlights with extra batteries
- ☐ Cell phone with charger, extra battery and solar charger
- ☐ Whistle to signal for help
- ☐ Local maps
- ☐ Pet supplies
- ☐ Baby supplies
- ☐ Books, games or puzzles
- ☐ A favorite stuffed animal or blanket

Remember, traffic lights will not work!

Figure 44.2. Emergency Kit Checklist for Kids *(Source: "Emergency Kit Checklist for Kids," U.S. Fire Administration (USFA).)*

Chapter 45

Gardening Health and Safety Tips

This chapter offer tips to help keep you safe and healthy so that you can enjoy the beauty and bounty gardening can bring.

Dress to Protect

Gear up to protect yourself from lawn and garden pests, harmful chemicals, sharp or motorized equipment, insects, and the harmful rays of too much sun.

- Wear safety goggles, sturdy shoes, and long pants to prevent injury when using power tools and equipment.

- Protect your hearing when using machinery. If you have to raise your voice to talk to someone who is an arm's length away, the noise can be potentially harmful to your hearing.

- Wear gloves to lower the risk for skin irritations, cuts, and certain contaminants.

- Use insect repellent containing N, N-diethyl-meta-toluamide (DEET). Protect yourself from diseases caused by mosquitoes and ticks. Wear long-sleeved shirts, and tuck your pants into your socks. You may also want to wear high rubber boots since ticks are usually located close to the ground.

- Lower your risk for sunburn and skin cancer. Wear long sleeves, wide-brimmed hats, sun shades, and sunscreen with a sun protective factor (SPF) of 15 or higher.

About This Chapter: This chapter includes text excerpted from "Gardening Health and Safety Tips," Centers for Disease Control and Prevention (CDC), December 23, 2015. Reviewed July 2019.

Know Your Limits in the Heat

Even being out for short periods of time in high temperatures can cause serious health problems. Monitor your activities and time in the sun to lower your risk for heat-related illness. If you are outside in hot weather for most of the day you will need to make an effort to drink more fluids. Eat healthy foods to help keep you energized. Avoid drinking liquids that contain alcohol or large amounts of sugar, especially in the heat. Take breaks often. Try to rest in shaded areas so that your body's thermostat will have a chance to recover. Stop working if you experience breathlessness or muscle soreness.

Put Safety First

Powered and unpowered tools and equipment can cause serious injury. Limit distractions, use chemicals and equipment properly, and be aware of hazards to lower your risk for injury.

- Follow instructions and warning labels on chemicals and lawn and garden equipment.

- Make sure the equipment is working properly.

- Sharpen tools carefully.

- Keep harmful chemicals, tools, and equipment out of children's reach.

Tips for Persons with Disabilities and Physical Activity

Talk to your healthcare provider if you have physical, mental, or environmental concerns that may impair your ability to work in the garden safely.

- If you have arthritis, use tools that are easy to grasp and that fit your ability. Research shows that two and a half hours per week of moderate physical activity can give you more energy and can help relieve arthritis pain and stiffness.

- If you are taking medications that may make you drowsy or impair your judgment or reaction time, do not operate machinery, climb ladders, or do activities that may increase your risk for injury.

- Listen to your body. Monitor your heart rate, level of fatigue, and physical discomfort.

- Call 911 if you get injured, experience chest and arm pain, dizziness, lightheadedness, or heat-related illness.

Enjoy the Benefits of Physical Activity

Gardening is an excellent way to get physical activity. Active people are less likely than inactive people to be obese or have high blood pressure, type 2 diabetes, osteoporosis, heart disease, stroke, depression, colon cancer, and premature death.

- Be active for at least two and a half hours a week. Include activities that raise your breathing and heart rates and that strengthen your muscles. Help kids and teens be active for at least one hour a day.

- If you have been inactive, start out with just a few minutes of physical activity each day. Gradually build up time and intensity.

- Vary your gardening activities to keep your interest and to broaden the range of benefits.

Get Vaccinated

Vaccinations can prevent many diseases and save lives. All adults should get a tetanus vaccination every 10 years. Tetanus lives in the soil and enters the body through breaks in the skin. Because gardeners use sharp tools, dig in the dirt, and handle plants with sharp points, they are particularly prone to tetanus infections.

- Before you start gardening, make sure your tetanus/diphtheria (Td) vaccination is up to date.

- Ask your healthcare provider if you need any other vaccinations.

Chapter 46

What Working Teens Need to Know about Safety

You are earning your own money. You are making new friends. You are learning new things and becoming independent. Work can be a fun, rewarding, and exciting part of your life. But, did you know that your job could harm you? Every nine minutes, a U.S. teen gets hurt on the job. It does not have to be this way. You have a right to be safe and healthy at work.

> Young workers have high rates of job-related injury. These injuries are often the result of the many hazards present in the places they typically work, such as sharp knives and slippery floors in restaurants. Limited or no prior work experience and a lack of safety training also contribute to high injury rates. Middle and high school workers may be at increased risk for injury since they may not have the strength or cognitive ability needed to perform certain job duties.
>
> *(Source: "Young Worker Safety and Health," Centers for Disease Control and Prevention (CDC).)*

Safe Work for Young Workers

Safe work is rewarding work. Your employer has a responsibility to provide a safe workplace. Employers must follow all the Occupational Safety and Health Administration (OSHA) safety and health standards to prevent you from being injured or becoming ill on the job. If you are under 18 years of age, there may be limits on the hours you work, the jobs you do, and the equipment you use.

About This Chapter: Text in this chapter begins with excerpts from "Are You a Teen Worker?" Centers for Disease Control and Prevention (CDC), March 2012. Reviewed July 2019; Text under the heading "Safe Work for Young Workers" is excerpted from "Young Workers," Occupational Safety and Health Administration (OSHA), May 10, 2012. Reviewed July 2019.

You Have Rights at Work

You have the right to:

- Work in a safe place

- Receive safety and health training in a language that you understand

- Ask questions if you do not understand instructions or if something seems unsafe

- Use and be trained on required safety gear, such as hard hats, goggles, and earplugs

- Exercise your workplace safety rights without retaliation or discrimination

- File a confidential complaint with OSHA if you believe there is a serious hazard or that your employer is not following OSHA standards

Your Employer Has Responsibilities

Your employer must:

- Provide a workplace free from serious recognized hazards, and follow all OSHA safety and health standards

- Provide training about workplace hazards and required safety gear

- Tell you where to get answers to your safety or health questions

- Tell you what to do if you get hurt on the job

Employers must pay for most types of safety gear.

Ways to Stay Safe on the Job

To help protect yourself, you can:

- Report unsafe conditions to a shift/team leader or supervisor

- Wear any safety gear required to do your job

- Follow the safety rules

- Ask questions.

- Ask for help, if needed

Part Five
Outdoor and Recreation Safety

Chapter 47

Sports and Exercise Safety

Playing sports can be fun, but it can also be dangerous if you are not careful. You can help prevent injuries by:

- Getting a physical to make sure you are healthy before you start playing your sport

- Wearing the right shoes, gear, and equipment

- Drinking lots of water

- Warming up and stretching

If you have already hurt yourself playing a sport, make sure you recover completely before you start up again. If possible, protect the injured part of your body with padding, a brace, or special equipment. When you do start playing again, start slowly.

Safety in Sports
Stay in the game with these tips:

- If you are new to a sport, work your way up slowly.
- Before you start a sport, see your doctor for a sports' physical.
- Follow safety rules for your sport.

About This Chapter: Text in this chapter begins with excerpts from "Sports Safety," MedlinePlus, National Institutes of Health (NIH), December 28, 2016; Text under the heading "Physical Activity Safety Tips" is excerpted from "Physical Activity Safety Tips for Girls," girlshealth.gov, Office on Women's Health (OWH), March 27, 2015. Reviewed July 2019.

- Talk to your coach about any safety concerns, or ask your parent or guardian to talk to your coach.

- Give your body a break. Experts suggest to take at least one day off per week from your sport or training schedule and at least two to three months off from your sport each year.

- If you train a lot in a high-impact sport, such as running, try replacing some intense training with lower-impact activities, such as biking.

- Try different sports. Playing the same sport over and over can put repeated stress on certain parts of your body.

- Strengthen your muscles. Conditioning exercises, such as sit-ups and push-ups, can strengthen the muscles you use when you compete.

- Skip special supplements. Products may claim to help you lose weight, bulk up, or improve your performance. Often these do not work, and they can even hurt you. Remember, all you really need to succeed is good nutrition.

(Source: "Playing Sports," girlshealth.gov, Office on Women's Health (OWH).)

Physical Activity Safety Tips

Take these basic steps to stay safe:

- **Being active** can be great for you and great fun—but not if you get hurt. Stay smart, safe, and strong.

- **Be active regularly.** Being active regularly builds fitness, and fit folks have a lower chance of getting hurt.

- **Build up slowly.** Pick activities you can do now, and then slowly challenge yourself. You might increase how often you are active or how long you are active each time. For example, maybe add five minutes to your workout every week or two.

- **Value variety.** Try to do a mix of activities so you do not put too much strain on the same parts of your body all the time.

- **Be careful on hot or humid days.** If possible, move your exercise indoors. That is also a good idea on days with a lot of air pollution. If you are going to be outside, rest in the shade, take breaks, and drink lots of water.

- **Drink plenty of fluids.** You need to drink before, during, and after activity.

- **Find safe places.** Try to stay away from traffic and dark areas, for example. And avoid places with a lot of holes or other things that could make you fall.

- **Follow the rules of the game.** Remember that many of the rules were made to keep you safe.

- **Always use the right safety equipment.** Make sure that your safety gear fits right and is in good shape.

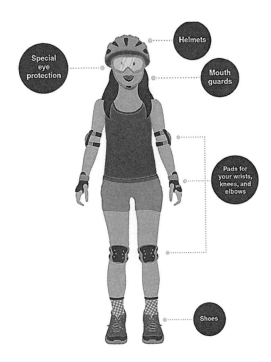

Figure 47.1. Safety Equipment

From helmets to shoes, the right equipment can help keep you safe when playing sports or being active.

Chapter 48

Safe Bicycling

There were 783 bicyclists killed in traffic crashes in the United States in 2017. As you might expect, when a crash occurs between a vehicle and a bike, it is the cyclist who is most likely to be injured. In this chapter, you will learn bicycle safety tips and rules of the road, from properly fitting your helmet to driving defensively and predictably. Find out what you can do to prevent bicycle injuries and deaths, and remember that a large percentage of crashes can be avoided if motorists and cyclists follow the rules of the road and watch out for each other.

Bicycle Safety

Americans are increasingly bicycling to commute, for exercise, or just for fun. By law, bicycles on the roadway are vehicles with the same rights and responsibilities as motorized vehicles.

Helmets

Every bike ride begins with putting on a helmet. But, it is equally important that you ensure a proper fit so your helmet can best protect you.

Size can vary between manufacturers. Follow the steps to fit a helmet properly. It may take time to ensure a proper helmet fit, but your life is worth it. It is usually easier to look in the mirror or have someone else adjust the straps.

About This Chapter: This chapter includes text excerpted from "Bicycle Safety," National Highway Traffic Safety Administration (NHTSA), November 7, 2018.

How Can You Tell Which Helmet Is the Right One to Use?

There are safety standards for most types of helmets. Bicycle and motorcycle helmets must comply with mandatory federal safety standards. Helmets for many other recreational activities are subject to voluntary safety standards. Helmets that meet the requirements of a mandatory or voluntary safety standard are designed and tested to protect the user from receiving a skull fracture or severe brain injury while wearing the helmet. The protection that the appropriate helmet can provide is dependent upon achieving a proper fit and wearing it correctly; for many activities, chin straps are specified in the standard, and they are essential for the helmet to function properly. For example, the bicycle standard requires that chin straps be strong enough to keep the helmet on the head and in the proper position during a fall or collision.

(Source: "Which Helmet for Which Activity?" U.S. Consumer Product Safety Commission (CPSC).)

Avoid Crashes
Decreasing Risk of Crashes

There are two main types of crashes: the most common (falls) and the most serious (the ones with cars). Regardless of the reason for the crash, prevention is the name of the game. There are things you can do to decrease your risk of a crash. First, know some bicycle safety facts:

- Regardless of the season, bicyclist deaths occurred most often between 6 p.m. and 9 p.m.

- Bicyclist deaths occurred most often in urban areas (75%) when compared to rural areas (25%) in 2017.

- Bicyclist deaths were 8 times higher for males than females in 2017.

- Alcohol was involved in 37 percent of all fatal bicyclist crashes in 2017.

Ride responsibly, and remember that all states require bicyclists on the roadway to follow the same rules and responsibilities as motorists.

Be Prepared before Heading Out

- Ride a bike that fits you. If it is too big, it is harder to control the bike.

- Ride a bike that works. It really does not matter how well you ride if the brakes do not work.

- Wear equipment to protect you and make you more visible to others, such as a bike helmet, bright clothing (during the day), reflective gear, and a white front light and red rear light, and reflectors on your bike (at night, or when visibility is poor).

- Ride one per seat, with both hands on the handlebars, unless signaling a turn.

- Carry all items in a backpack or strapped to the back of the bike.

- Tuck and tie your shoelaces and pant legs so they do not get caught in your bike chain.

- Plan your route. If driving as a vehicle on the road, choose routes with less traffic and slower speeds. Your safest route may be away from traffic altogether, in a bike lane or on a bike path.

Drive Defensively—Focused and Alert

Be focused and alert to the road and all traffic around you; anticipate what others may do, before they do it. This is defensive driving—the quicker you notice a potential conflict, the quicker you can act to avoid a potential crash:

- Drive with the flow, in the same direction as traffic.

- Obey street signs, signals, and road markings, just like a car.

- Assume the other person does not see you; look ahead for hazards or situations to avoid that may cause you to fall, such as toys, pebbles, potholes, grates, train tracks.

- No texting, listening to music, or using anything that distracts you by taking your eyes and ears or your mind off the road and traffic.

Drive Predictably

By driving predictably, motorists get a sense of what you intend to do and can react to avoid a crash.

Drive where you are expected to be seen, travel in the same direction as traffic, and signal and look over your shoulder before changing lane position or turning.

Avoid or minimize sidewalk riding. Cars do not expect to see moving traffic on a sidewalk and do not look for you when backing out of a driveway or turning. Sidewalks sometimes end unexpectedly, forcing the bicyclist into the road when a car is not expecting to look for a bicyclist. If you must ride on the sidewalk remember to:

- Check your law to make sure sidewalk riding is legal.

- Watch for pedestrians.

- Pass pedestrians with care by first announcing "on your left" or "passing on your left," or use a bell.

- Ride in the same direction as traffic. This way, if the sidewalk ends, you are already riding with the flow of traffic. If crossing a street, motorists will look left, right, left for traffic. When you are to the driver's left, the driver is more likely to see you.

- Slow and look for traffic (left-right-left and behind) when crossing a street from a sidewalk; be prepared to stop and follow the pedestrian signals.

- Slow down and look for cars backing out of driveways or turning.

Improve Your Riding Skills

No one learns to drive a vehicle safely without practice and experience; safely riding your bike in traffic requires the same preparation. Start by riding your bike in a safe environment away from traffic (a park, path, or empty parking lot).

Take an on-bike class through your school, recreation department, local bike shop, or bike advocacy group. Confidence in traffic comes with learning how to navigate and communicate with other drivers, bicyclists, and pedestrians. Reviewing and practicing as a safe pedestrian or bicyclist is great preparation for safe riding.

Drivers: Share the Road

People on bicycles have the same rights and responsibilities as people behind the wheel of a vehicle.

- Yield to bicyclists as you would motorists, and do not underestimate their speed. This will help avoid turning in front of a bicyclist traveling on the road or sidewalk, often at an intersection or driveway.

- In parking lots, at stop signs, when packing up, or when parking, search your surroundings for other vehicles, including bicycles.

- Drivers turning right on red should look to the right and behind to avoid hitting a bicyclist approaching from the right rear. Stop completely, and look left-right-left and behind before turning right on red.

- Obey the speed limit, reduce speed for road conditions, and drive defensively to avoid a crash with a cyclist.

- Give cyclists room. Do not pass them too closely. Pass bicyclists as you would any other vehicle—when it is safe to move over into an adjacent lane.

Chapter 49

Water Sports Safety

What do surfing, fishing, water skiing, and swimming have in common? They are all a lot of fun, and they all take place in, on, or around the water. Water activities are a great way to stay cool and have a good time with your friends or your family. Take along these tips—and your common sense—to get wet, make waves, and have a blast.

Tips for Water Sports Safety

- **Do learn to swim.** If you like to have a good time doing water activities, being a strong swimmer is a must.

- **Do take a friend along.** Even though you may be a good swimmer, you never know when you may need help. Having friends around is safer and more fun.

- **Do know your limits.** Watch out for the "too's"—too tired, too cold, too far from safety, too much sun, too much hard activity.

- **Do swim in supervised (watched) areas only,** and follow all signs and warnings.

- **Do wear a life jacket** when boating, jet skiing, water skiing, rafting, or fishing.

- **Do stay alert to currents.** They can change quickly. If you get caught in a strong current, do not fight it. Swim parallel to the shore until you have passed through it. Near piers, jetties (lines of big rocks), small dams, and docks, the current gets unpredictable and could knock you around. If you find it hard to move around, head to shore. Learn

About This Chapter: This chapter includes text excerpted from "BAM! Body and Mind—H_2O Smarts," Centers for Disease Control and Prevention (CDC), May 9, 2015. Reviewed July 2019.

to recognize and watch for dangerous waves and signs of rip currents—water that is a weird color, really choppy, foamy, or filled with pieces of stuff.

- **Do keep an eye on the weather.** If you spot bad weather (dark clouds, lighting), pack up and take the fun inside.

- **Do not mess around in the water.** Pushing or dunking your friends can easily get out of hand.

- **Do not dive into shallow water.** If you do not know how deep the water is, do not dive.

- **Do not float where you cannot swim.** Keep checking to see if the water is too deep or if you are too far away from the shore or the poolside.

Water Wisdom

Icy

If the water is cold, a wet suit can be your best friend. Wearing it will make you feel more comfortable, and you will keep your body temperature from dropping to the danger zone.

Floaters versus Personal Flotation Device

Q: Can blow-up objects, such as rafts, work as life preservers?

A: Nope. Although they float, they will not do the trick.

Did You Know?

Water covers 80 percent of the Earth!

Lifeline

If you see someone struggling in the water, go get help. You can also throw out a life preserver or another object that floats, but do not jump in yourself. If you jump in without anyone else around, who will help save you if there is a problem?

Watch out for Mother Nature

Even if you are an expert, things that you cannot control can get you into trouble. Look out for signs warning you that the water is not clean because polluted water could make you sick.

It is also smart to keep clear of objects such as plants and animals that are in the water. They can cause problems for you, so go the other way if you see them.

Finally, if you are outside, you need to guard against the sun. Those burning rays reflect off the water and sand onto you, and they can really spoil the fun. So, rub on some sunscreen to get sunproof.

The Deal on Water Parks

If you have ever been to a water park, you know that they are so much fun.

Need-to-knows for having a great time on ride after ride are as follows:

- Read all the signs before going on a ride. Make sure you are tall enough and old enough. Ask questions if you are not sure about how you are supposed to go on the ride. (On most water slides, you should go down face up, arms crossed behind your head, and feet first with your ankles crossed.)

- When you go from ride to ride, do not run. It is slippery.

- Bumping into others on a slide can hurt. That is why no "chains" of people are allowed on water rides. So, count five seconds after the rider ahead of you has gone before you take your turn.

- Wear a life preserver; the park supplies it for a reason.

The Deal on Boating and Jet Skiing

Skimming over the water is a great ride. You probably are not driving a boat or jet ski yourself just yet, but they are lots of fun to ride with an adult. You and your parents can check the state rules for how old you have to be.

Stay alert! When you are riding, keep a lookout for other boats, jet skiers, water skiers, divers, and swimmers. Who has the right-of-way? Generally, drivers should keep to their right when they are passing other boats—just like you do when you are walking in the hall at school.

Always ride at a speed that will let you stay in control so you can stop or go another way if you need to. It is also not a good idea to jump wakes (tracks in the water left by other boats or jet skis) or speed through choppy water because it is easy to lose control.

Do not ride with a driver who has been drinking alcohol.

Make sure you know and practice what to do if someone falls out of the boat.

Some people teak surf (hold on to the back of the boat and then let go to ride the wave that the boat makes), but you should not copy them. Teak surfers get too close to the boat, do not wear life jackets, and breathe exhaust fumes (chemicals) that the boat makes.

Chapter 50

All-Terrain Vehicles

Over the past 30 years, all-terrain vehicles (ATVs) have grown increasingly popular recreationally, and they have become a valuable asset at work. With an estimated 11 million in use in 2010 for both work and recreation, ATVs have become a common means of transportation.

All-terrain vehicles were first manufactured in the late 1960s as farm-to-town vehicles for use in isolated, mountainous areas in Japan. They were first introduced in the United States for agricultural applications in the early 1980s. ATVs have many unique features that enable them to operate in a variety of harsh environments where other larger, less mobile vehicles cannot be used, making them very useful in the workplace. Oversized and low pressure (4 to 5 psi) tires, low weight (600 to 1000 pounds), and easy maneuverability make ATVs ideal in many work settings. ATVs are commonly used by workers in border patrol and security, construction operations, emergency medical response, search and rescue, law enforcement, land management and surveying, military operations, mineral and oil exploration, pipeline maintenance, ranching and farming, small-scale forestry activities, and wildland fire control, among others. Farmers and other landowners have described ATVs as filling a valuable niche between a truck and a tractor. Since licensing and training requirements vary widely by state, many companies conduct their own training or use the resources available to public and private organizations from the ATV Safety Institute, a nonprofit division of the Specialty Vehicle Institute of America (SVIA).

About This Chapter: This chapter includes text excerpted from "All-Terrain Vehicles and Work," Centers for Disease Control and Prevention (CDC), August 31, 2017.

What the Data Tell Us
Economic Cost of Deaths

A review of 129 ATV-related occupational deaths from 2003 to 2006 indicated that the collective lifetime societal cost of these deaths was $103.6 million, with an average cost of $803,100 per death. In the western United States, 11 states accounted for over 60 percent of the deaths, with 4 states (Montana, Texas, Colorado, and South Dakota) accounting for nearly one-third of all work-related ATV deaths during the 4-year period. Nearly two-thirds of the deaths were to workers in agricultural production at a cost of $62.3 million.

What You Can Do to Ensure Safe Use of All-Terrain Vehicles

All-terrain vehicles can be used safely if used properly, the risks are understood, and precautions are taken to reduce the likelihood of injury. The recommendations listed below should be followed to ensure safe operation of ATVs:

- Wear a helmet, eye protection, long shirts and pants, sturdy boots, and gloves.

- Participate in hands-on training in the safe handling and operation of an ATV.

- Conduct a preride inspection of the tires, brakes, headlights, etc., and follow the manufacturer's recommendations for the safe use of the ATV.

- Understand how implements and attachments may affect the stability and handling of the ATV.

- Never exceed the manufacturer's specified hauling and towing capacity or weight limits, and ensure that any cargo is balanced, secured, and correctly loaded on the racks provided.

- Be aware of potential hazards, such as trees, ruts, rocks, streams, and gullies, and follow the hazard warnings posted.

- Drive at speeds safe for the weather and terrain, and never operate ATVs on surfaces not designed for ATVs, such as paved roads and highways.

- Never permit passengers on the ATV, unless the ATV has an additional seat specifically designed to carry them.

- Never operate an ATV while under the influence of drugs or alcohol.

Children and young people under the age of 16 should not ride adult ATVs.

All ATV users should take a hands-on safety training course.

Always wear a helmet and safety gear such as boots and gloves while on an ATV.

Never drive an ATV on paved roads. Never drive while under the influence of drugs or alcohol.

Never drive a youth or single-rider adult ATV with a passenger, and never ride these vehicles as a passenger. There are some ATVs that are designed for two riders. Passengers on tandem ATVs should be at least 12 years old.

Figure 50.1. All-Terrain Vehicle Safety Tips *(Source: "All-Terrain Vehicle Safety," U.S. Consumer Product Safety Commission (CPSC).)*

Chapter 51

Snowmobile Safety

Snowmobile use is dependent on weather conditions; winters with greater snowfalls and lower temperatures allow persons more opportunity to use snowmobiles. A study has found that snowmobile-related fatalities has been growing over the years. The results of the study indicate that the primary causes of these fatalities were excessive speed, inattentive or careless operation, and inexperience.

Efforts to reduce snowmobile fatalities should focus on improving safety measures, including establishing speed limits, strengthening enforcement of snowmobile operating rules, and promoting safety education. Strengthening enforcement of existing laws and increasing safety measures might reduce fatalities associated with snowmobiles. State and local officials should consider enacting additional measures to promote safety, especially those aimed at reducing speed on trails and educating operators on more cautious and attentive use of snowmobiles.

Safety Tips for Recreational Snowmobiling

The U.S. Consumer Product Safety Commission (CPSC) recommends the following safety tips for recreational snowmobiling:

- Never drive your snowmobile alone or on unfamiliar ground. Have someone ride along with you, so you can help each other in case of breakdown or accident.

About This Chapter: Text in this chapter begins with excerpts from "Snowmobile Fatalities—Maine, New Hampshire, and Vermont, 2002–2003," Centers for Disease Control and Prevention (CDC), December 19, 2003. Reviewed July 2019; Text under the heading "Safety Tips for Recreational Snowmobiling" is excerpted from "Snowmobile Hazards," U.S. Consumer Product Safety Commission (CPSC), February 1, 2001. Reviewed July 2019.

- Drive only on established and marked trails or in areas open to snowmobiles.

- Avoid waterways. Frozen lakes and rivers can be fatal. It is almost impossible to judge adequate ice coverage or depth.

- Avoid driving in bad weather. Check warnings for snow, ice and wind chill conditions before starting.

- Watch the path ahead to avoid rocks, trees, fences (particularly barbed wire), ditches, and other obstacles.

- Slow down at the top of a hill. A cliff, snow bank or other unforeseen hazard could be on the other side. Do not hurdle snow banks. You have control only when your skis are on the ground.

- Do not wear headphones or earbuds while snowmobiling.

- Wear a snowmobile helmet that meets safety standards DOT FMVSS 218 or Snell M2010 or ECE 22.05.

- Learn the snowmobile traffic laws and regulations for the area. Many states prohibit snowmobiles on public roads. Some states have minimum age requirements for drivers.

- Be sensible about stopping at roads or railroad tracks. Signal your turns to other drivers. Avoid tailgating. Control speed according to conditions.

- Use extra caution if driving at night, because unseen obstacles could be fatal. Do not drive faster than your headlights will allow you to see. Wear reflective clothing. Do not open new trails after dark.

- Never drink while driving your snowmobile. Drinking and driving can prove fatal.

- Be sure the snowmobile is properly maintained and in good operating condition.

Why Are Helmets So Important?

For many recreational activities, wearing a helmet can reduce the risk of a severe head injury and even save your life. During a typical fall or collision, much of the impact energy is absorbed by the helmet, rather than your head and brain.

(Source: "Which Helmet for Which Activity?" U.S. Consumer Product Safety Commission (CPSC).)

Chapter 52

Skating, Skateboarding, and Snow Skiing

Inline Skating
Gear Up

There are several different types of inline skates, depending on the type of skating you do. Recreational skates have a plastic boot and four wheels. These skates are best for beginners. Hockey skates have laces and are made of leather with small wheels for quick movement. Racing skates have five wheels and, usually, no brake. Freestyle skates have three wheels and a pick stop for tricks. Fitness skates have larger wheels and are used for cross-training. Aggressive skates, the kind worn by X Games competitors, are made of thick plastic with small wheels for quick movement and grind plates to protect the skate when doing tricks. No matter what kind of skates you wear, always wear a helmet, as well as wrist guards, elbow pads, and knee pads.

Play It Safe

Avoid getting hurt by making sure that your helmet and pads are on correctly. Your helmet should be tightly buckled, with the front coming down to right over your eyebrow, and your pads should be on tight so that they do not slip while you are skating. It is also important that your helmet is approved by one of the groups who test helmets to see which ones are the best: the Consumer Product Safety Commission (CPSC) or Snell B-95 standards are best for inline

About This Chapter: This chapter includes text excerpted from "BAM! Body and Mind—Activity Information Sheets," Centers for Disease Control and Prevention (CDC), April 30, 2018.

skating helmets. Make sure you are always in control of your speed, turns, and stops, and be careful of cracks in the pavement where you are skating—they can be dangerous if your wheels get caught in them. It is best to go skating out of the way of traffic and other people (skating rinks are great places to skate).

How to Play

If you are just beginning inline skating, here are some tips to get you rolling.

Practice balancing on your skates by walking in them on a flat, grassy area. As you move to the pavement, balance yourself without trying to move. Gradually begin to skate by moving forward, but do not go too fast. Keep your knees bent and flexible when you skate—it will keep you more stable. And if you fall, fall forward. Then you will fall on your knee pads—they are there to protect you.

It is also a good idea to take lessons from a certified instructor; you can find one through the International Inline Skating Association (IISA). As you get more skilled on your skates, there are several types of competitive inline skating activities, such as speed skating and aggressive skating, which includes events such as those at the X Games. There are also sports leagues just for those who play on wheels, such as roller hockey, roller soccer, and roller basketball.

As might be expected, at least half of all roller-skating injuries are suffered by teenagers, and well over two-thirds of the injuries were to girls and women. By contrast, the great majority of skateboard accidents occurred to boys and men. Many of these serious injuries might have been avoided if the roller skaters knew the proper way to fall. Typically, when skaters lose their balance, they try to break their fall in ways which increase the likelihood of fractures and sprains, such as falling forward onto outstretched arms. Some of these bruises and broken bones can be avoided if skaters follow these safety tips:

- Wear protective padding on elbows and knees.
- Try to fall in a relaxed rather than stiffened posture.
- When falling, try to land on flesh or muscle rather than on bones or joints.
- Try to skate on smooth surfaces, and keep watch for stones, twigs, broken cement or other surface irregularities.

(Source: "Roller Skates Pass Skateboards as Major Cause of Recreational Injury," U.S. Consumer Product Safety Commission (CPSC).)

Skateboarding
Gear Up

Skateboards can be bought preassembled, or you can buy all of the pieces and put it together yourself. Preassembled boards are best for beginners, until you decide if skateboarding is really for you. If you are putting your own board together, you will need a deck (the board itself), grip tape for the top of the deck so your feet do not slip, two trucks (the metal parts that are the axles of the wheels), four wheels, and two bearings per wheel (these keep the wheels spinning on the truck's axle). Before each time you ride, make sure your trucks are tightened and your wheels are spinning properly. Do not forget to wear a helmet, knee and elbow pads, and wrist guards. It is important that your helmet is approved by one of the groups who test helmets to see which ones are the best: the Snell B-95 standard is best for skateboarding helmets. Nonslippery shoes are a good idea too, so you can have better control of your board.

Play It Safe

Before you ride, make sure you give your board a safety check to make sure everything is put together right. Always wear all of your protective gear, including a helmet, knee and elbow pads, and wrist guards. If you do tricks with your board, you may also want to wear gloves to protect your hands from the pavement. If you are just starting out, skate on a smooth, flat surface so you can practice keeping control of your board. And no matter how experienced you are, never hold on to the back of a moving vehicle. It is best to skate out of the way of traffic and other people (skate parks are great places to skate). But, if you are skating in streets near your house, be aware of cars and people around you, and stay out of their way. Also, once the sun sets, it is a good idea to put up your board for the night because skating in the dark can be dangerous.

Snow Skiing

If you think you are too young to learn how to ski, think again.

Gear Up

Skis. Are your skis the right size? If the tip of your upright ski reaches your face between your nose and chin, they are. If you are a beginner, shorter skis will be easier to control. The bindings (the part that holds your boot to the ski) are the most important parts of the ski; to make sure they do not break, get them tested regularly by a pro.

Make sure your boots fit and are comfortable. In general, ski boots are ½ size smaller than your normal shoe size.

Ski helmets. Be a trendsetter by picking up the helmet habit. Choose an American Society for Testing and Materials (ASTM)-approved model that fits right, is ventilated, and does not affect your hearing or field of vision.

Ski poles are used to give you balance, to help you get up if you fall, or if you need to side-step up a hill.

Goggles are important to protect your eyes from flying dirt or snow, as well as stopping the sun's glare while going down the slopes. Some goggles come with fun tinted lenses. If you do not have goggles, you can use sunglasses instead.

If you are renting equipment, the staff at the ski shop can help you find all the right stuff.

Stay Warm on the Slopes

- Long underwear to keep you warm and absorb sweat

- Insulated tops and pants, such as sweaters and leggings. This layer should be warm but not baggy.

- Ski pants and jackets to protect you from snow and wetness

- A hat. 60 percent of heat loss is through the head.

Play It Safe

If you can, sign up for lessons from a ski school, even if you have taken lessons before; your instructor can teach you all the right moves, for beginners, as well as for more advanced students.

The key to skiing is control of your equipment and your speed. If you feel yourself start to lose control, fall onto your backside or your side, and do not attempt to get up until you stop sliding.

The easiest way to get hurt while skiing is to try a run or a move that is too hard. Always ski on trails that match your skill level, and never attempt a jumping move or another trick unless taught by an instructor.

Did you know that it is just as important to drink water when you are active in the cold as in the heat? Why? Higher altitudes and colder air can cause your body to lose water. If you experience dizziness or have a dry mouth, headache, or muscle cramps, take a water break. A good rule would be to drink water or a sports drinks before, during, and after your ski runs.

Always check the snow conditions of the slope before you go up; you will need to ski differently in icy conditions than you would if you were on wet snow or in deep powder.

Altitude can zap your energy. Do not push it. Ski the easier runs later in the day when you are tired. Most importantly, know when to quit.

While on the slopes, set a meeting time and place to check in with your parents or friends, and always ski with a buddy. And wear plenty of sunblocks because those rays are strong on the mountain due to the high altitude and reflection off the snow.

Be sure to keep the responsibility code for skiers in mind:

- Always stay in control, and be able to stop or avoid other people or objects.

- People ahead of you have the right of way. It is your responsibility to avoid them.

- Do not stop where you obstruct a trail or are not visible from above.

- Whenever starting downhill or merging into a trail, look uphill and yield to others.

- Always use devices to help prevent runaway equipment.

- Observe all posted signs and warnings. Keep off closed trails and out of closed areas.

- Before using any lift, you must have the knowledge and ability to load, ride, and unload safely.

- Finally, watch out for the sun. Wear a t-shirt and sunscreen to make sure you do not get sunburned.

Part Six
Emergency and Disaster Preparedness

Chapter 53

Making a Disaster Plan

Make a plan today. Your family may not be together if a disaster strikes, so it is important to know which types of disasters could affect your area. Know how you will contact one another and reconnect if separated. Establish a family meeting place that is familiar and easy to find.

Preparing for a disaster can reduce the fear, anxiety, and losses that disasters cause. A disaster can be a natural disaster, such as a hurricane, tornado, flood or earthquake. It might also be human-made, such as a bioterrorist attack or chemical spill. You should know the risks and danger signs of different types of disasters. You should also have a disaster plan. Be ready to evacuate your home, and know how to treat basic medical problems. Make sure you have the insurance you need, including special types, such as flood insurance.

(Source: "Disaster Preparation and Recovery," MedlinePlus, National Institutes of Health (NIH).)

Step 1: Put together a plan by discussing these four questions with your family, friends, or household to start your emergency plan.

- How will I receive emergency alerts and warnings?

- What is my shelter plan?

- What is my evacuation route?

- What is my family/household communication plan?

About This Chapter: This chapter includes text excerpted from "Make a Plan," Ready, U.S. Department of Homeland Security (DHS), July 19, 2017.

Step 2: Consider specific needs in your household. As you prepare your plan, tailor your plans and supplies to your specific daily living needs and responsibilities. Discuss your needs and responsibilities and how people in the network can assist each other with communication; caring for any children; business; pets; or specific needs, such as the operation of durable medical equipment. Create your own personal network for specific areas where you need assistance. Keep in mind some of these factors when developing your plan:

- Different ages of members within your household

- Responsibilities for assisting others

- Locations frequented

- Dietary needs

- Medical needs, including prescriptions and equipment

- Disabilities or access and functional needs, including devices and equipment

- Languages spoken

- Cultural and religious considerations

- Pets or service animals

- Households with school-aged children

Step 3: Create and fill out a family emergency plan.

Step 4: Practice your plan with your family/household.

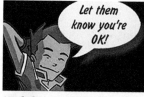 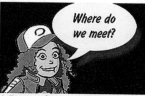 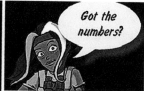

* Pick the same person for each family member to call or email. It might be easier to reach someone who's out of town.
* Text, don't talk, unless it's an emergency. It may be easier to send a text, if you have a phone, and you don't want to tie up phone lines for emergency workers.

* Create a fire escape plan that has two ways out of every room and practice it twice a year.
* Choose a meeting spot near your home, then practice getting there.
* Choose a spot outside of your neighborhood in case you can't get home. Practice getting there from school, your friends' houses, and after school activities.

* Keep your family's contact info and meeting spot location in your backpack, wallet, or taped inside your school notebook. Put it in your cell phone if you have one.

Figure 53.1. Call a Family Meeting and Make a Plan

Types of Disasters
Be Informed

While flooding can happen at any time, floods can result from rain or melting snow, making them common in the spring. Flooding is a temporary overflow of water onto land that is normally dry. Floods are the most common natural disaster in the United States. Failing to evacuate flooded areas, entering floodwaters, or remaining after a flood has passed can result in injury or death.

Know what disasters and hazards could affect your area, how to get emergency alerts, and where you would go if you and your family need to evacuate. The following is a list of disasters and hazards that could affect your area:

- Active shooter

- Attacks in public places

- Bioterrorism

- Chemical emergencies

- Cybersecurity

- Drought

- Earthquakes

- Emergency alerts

- Explosions

- Extreme heat

- Floods

- Hazardous materials incidents

- Home fires

- Household chemical emergencies

- Hurricanes

- Landslides and debris flow

- Nuclear explosion

- Nuclear power plants

- Pandemic

- Power outages

- Radiological dispersion device

- Severe weather

- Snowstorms and extreme cold

- Space weather

- Thunderstorms and lightning

- Tornadoes

- Tsunamis

- Volcanoes

- Wildfires

No matter what kind of disaster you experience, it causes emotional distress. After a disaster, recovery can take time. Stay connected to your family and friends during this period.

(Source: "Disaster Preparation and Recovery," MedlinePlus, National Institutes of Health (NIH).)

Chapter 54

Building a Disaster Kit

Make sure your emergency kit is stocked with the items on the checklist below. Most of the items are inexpensive and easy to find, and any one of them could save your life. Headed to the store? Take a printout of the list. Once you take a look at the basic items, consider what unique needs your family might have, such as supplies for pets or seniors.

After an emergency, you may need to survive on your own for several days. Being prepared means having your own food, water, and other supplies to last for at least 72 hours. A disaster supplies kit is a collection of basic items your household may need in the event of an emergency.

Basic Disaster Supplies Kit

To assemble your kit, store items in airtight plastic bags and put your entire disaster supplies kit in one or two easy-to-carry containers, such as plastic bins or a duffel bag.

A basic emergency supply kit could include the following recommended items:

- Water—one gallon of water per person per day for at least three days, for drinking and sanitation

- Food—at least a three-day supply of nonperishable food

- Battery-powered or hand crank radio and a National Oceanic and Atmospheric Administration (NOAA) Weather Radio with a tone alert

About This Chapter: This chapter includes text excerpted from "Build a Kit," Ready, U.S. Department of Homeland Security (DHS), July 29, 2017.

- Flashlight

- First aid kit

- Extra batteries

- Whistle to signal for help

- Dust masks to help filter contaminated air

- Plastic sheeting and duct tape to shelter-in-place

- Moist towelettes, garbage bags, and plastic ties for personal sanitation

- Wrench or pliers to turn off utilities

- Manual can opener for food

- Local maps

- Cell phone with chargers and a backup battery

Additional Emergency Supplies

Consider adding the following items to your emergency supply kit based on your individual needs:

- Prescription medications

- Nonprescription medications, such as pain relievers, antidiarrheal medication, antacids, or laxatives

- Glasses and contact lens solution

- Infant formula, bottles, diapers, wipes, diaper rash cream

- Pet food and extra water for your pet

- Cash or traveler's checks

- Important family documents, such as copies of insurance policies, identification, and bank account records, saved electronically or in a waterproof, portable container

- Sleeping bag or warm blanket for each person

- Complete change of clothing that is appropriate for your climate and sturdy shoes

- Household chlorine bleach and medicine dropper to disinfect water

- Fire extinguisher

- Matches in a waterproof container

- Feminine supplies and personal hygiene items

- Mess kits, paper cups, plates, paper towels, and plastic utensils

- Paper and pencil

- Books, games, puzzles, or other activities for children

Maintaining Your Kit

After assembling your kit, remember to maintain it so it is ready when needed.

- Keep canned food in a cool, dry place.

- Store boxed food in a tightly closed plastic or metal containers.

- Replace expired items as needed.

- Rethink your needs every year, and update your kit as your family's needs change.

Kit Storage Locations

Since you do not know where you will be when an emergency occurs, prepare supplies for home, work, and vehicles.

- **Home:** Keep this kit in a designated place, and have it ready in case you have to leave your home quickly. Make sure all family members know where the kit is kept.

- **Work:** Be prepared to shelter at work for at least 24 hours. Your work kit should include food; water; and other necessities, such as medicines, as well as comfortable walking shoes that are stored in a "grab and go" case.

- **Vehicle:** In case you are stranded, keep a kit of emergency supplies in your car.

Chapter 55

Sheltering in Place: What It Means

Chemical, biological, or radiological contaminants may be released into the environment in such quantity and/or proximity to a place of business that it is safer to remain indoors rather than to evacuate. Such releases may be either accidental or intentional. Examples of situations that might result in a decision by you to institute "shelter-in-place" include an explosion in an ammonia refrigeration facility across the street, or a derailed and leaking tank car of chlorine on the rail line behind your home.

"Shelter-in-place" means selecting an interior room or rooms within your facility, or ones with no or few windows, and taking refuge there. In many cases, local authorities will issue advice to shelter-in-place via television (TV) or radio.

Get Inside, Stay Inside

If local officials tell you to stay put, act quickly. Listen carefully to local radio or television stations for instructions because the exact directions will depend on the emergency situation. In general, you should:

- Get inside. Bring your loved ones, your emergency supplies, and your pets, when possible.

- Find a safe spot in this location. The exact spot will depend on the type of emergency.

- Stay put in this location until officials say that it is safe to leave.

About This Chapter: Text in this chapter begins with excerpts from "Emergency Action Plan—Shelter-in-Place," Occupational Safety and Health Administration (OSHA), March 10, 2009. Reviewed July 2019; Text beginning with the heading "Get Inside, Stay Inside" is excerpted from "Stay Put—Learn How to Shelter in Place," Centers for Disease Control and Prevention (CDC), September 29, 2017.

Stay in Touch

Once you and your family are in place, let your emergency contact know what is happening and listen carefully for new information.

Call or text your emergency contact. Let them know where you are, if any family members are missing, and how you are doing.

Use your phone only as necessary. Keep the phone handy in case you need to report a life-threatening emergency. Otherwise, do not use the phone so that the lines will be available for emergency responders.

Keep listening to your radio, television, or phone for updates. Do not leave your shelter unless authorities tell you it is safe to do so. If they tell you to evacuate the area, follow their instructions.

Staying Put in Your Vehicle

In some emergencies, it is safer to pull over and stay in your car than to keep driving. If you are very close to home, your workplace, or a public building, go there immediately and go inside. Follow the "shelter in place" recommendations for that location. If you cannot get indoors quickly and safely:

- Pull over to the side of the road.

- Stop your vehicle in the safest place possible, and turn off the engine.

- If it is warm outside, it is better to stop under a bridge or in a shady spot so you do not get overheated.

- Stay where you are until officials say it is safe to get back on the road.

- Listen to the radio for updates and additional instructions.

- Modern car radios do not use much battery power, so listening to the radio for an hour or two should not cause your car battery to die.

- Even after it is safe to get back on the road, keep listening to the radio and follow the directions of law enforcement officials.

Mass Care Shelter

Even though mass care shelters often provide water, food, medicine and, basic sanitary facilities, you should plan to take your disaster supplies kit with you so you will have the supplies you require. Mass care sheltering can involve living with many people in a confined space, which can be difficult and unpleasant. To avoid conflicts in a stressful situation, it is important to cooperate with shelter managers and others assisting them. Keep in mind that alcoholic beverages and weapons are forbidden in emergency shelters and smoking is restricted.

Search for open shelters by texting SHELTER and a Zip Code to 43362.

(Source: "Shelter," Ready, U.S. Department of Homeland Security (DHS).)

Chapter 56

Things to Know about Tornados, Hurricanes, and Floods

About Tornados

Tornados can destroy buildings, flip cars, and create deadly flying debris. Tornados are a violently rotating column of air that extends from a thunderstorm to the ground. Tornados can:

- Happen anytime and anywhere
- Bring intense winds, over 200 miles per hour (MPH)
- Look like funnels

If you are under a tornado warning, find a safe shelter right away.

- If you can safely get to a sturdy building, then do so immediately.
- Go to a safe room, basement, or storm cellar.
- If you are in a building with no basement, then get to a small interior room on the lowest level.
- Stay away from windows, doors, and outside walls.
- Do not get under an overpass or bridge. You are safer in a low, flat location.

About This Chapter: Text under the heading "About Tornados" is excerpted from "Tornadoes," Ready, U.S, Department of Homeland Security (DHS), November 9, 2011. Reviewed July 2019; Text under the heading "About Hurricanes" is excerpted from "Hurricanes," Ready, U.S. Department of Homeland Security (DHS), June 6, 2018; Text under the heading "About Floods" is excerpted from "Floods," Ready, U.S. Department of Homeland Security (DHS), May 25, 2018.

- Watch out for flying debris that can cause injury or death.

- Use your arms to protect your head and neck.

How to Stay Safe When a Tornado Threatens
Prepare Now for a Tornado

- Know your area's tornado risk. In the United States, the Midwest and the Southeast have a greater risk for tornadoes.

- Know the signs of a tornado, including a rotating, funnel-shaped cloud; an approaching cloud of debris; or a loud roar—similar to a freight train.

- Sign up for your community's warning system. The Emergency Alert System (EAS) and the National Oceanic and Atmospheric Administration (NOAA) Weather Radio also provide emergency alerts. If your community has sirens, become familiar with the warning tone.

- Pay attention to weather reports. Meteorologists can predict when conditions might be right for a tornado.

- Identify and practice going to a safe shelter in the event of high winds, such as a safe room built using the Federal Emergency Management Agency (FEMA) criteria or a storm shelter built to the International Code Council (ICC) 500 standards. The next best protection is a small, interior, windowless room on the lowest level of a sturdy building.

- Consider constructing your own safe room that meets FEMA or ICC 500 standards.

Survive during a Tornado

- Immediately go to a safe location that you identified.

- Take additional cover by shielding your head and neck with your arms and putting materials such as furniture and blankets around you.

- Listen to the EAS, the NOAA Weather Radio, or local alerting systems for current emergency information and instructions.

- Do not try to outrun a tornado in a vehicle.

- If you are in a car or outdoors and cannot get to a building, cover your head and neck with your arms and cover your body with a coat or blanket, if possible.

Be Safe after a Tornado

- Keep listening to the EAS, the NOAA Weather Radio, and local authorities for updated information.

- If you are trapped, cover your mouth with a cloth or mask to avoid breathing in dust. Try to send a text, bang on a pipe or wall, or use a whistle instead of shouting.

- Stay clear of fallen power lines or broken utility lines.

- Do not enter damaged buildings until you are told that they are safe.

- Save your phone calls for emergencies. Phone systems are often down or busy after a disaster. Use text messaging or social media to communicate with family and friends.

- Be careful during cleanup. Wear thick-soled shoes, long pants, and work gloves.

About Hurricanes

Hurricanes are massive storm systems that form over warm ocean waters and move toward land. Potential threats from hurricanes include powerful winds, heavy rainfall, storm surges, coastal and inland flooding, rip currents, tornadoes, and landslides. The Atlantic hurricane season runs from June 1 to November 30. The Pacific hurricane season runs from May 15 to November 30. Hurricanes:

- Can happen along any U.S. coast or in any territory in the Atlantic or Pacific oceans

- Can affect areas more than 100 miles inland

- Are most active in September

If you are under a hurricane warning, find safe shelter right away.

- Determine how best to protect yourself from high winds and flooding.

  - Evacuate if you are told to do so.

  - Take refuge in a designated storm shelter or an interior room during high winds.

- Listen for emergency information and alerts.

- Only use generators outdoors and away from windows.

- Turn around; do not drown. Do not walk, swim, or drive through floodwaters.

How to Stay Safe When a Hurricane Threatens
Prepare Now for a Hurricane

- Know your area's risk of hurricanes.

- Sign up for your community's warning system. The EAS and NOAA Weather Radio also provide emergency alerts.

- If you are at risk for flash flooding, watch for warning signs, such as heavy rain.

- Practice going to a safe shelter, such as a FEMA safe room or an ICC 500 storm shelter, in the event of high winds. The next best protection is a small, interior, windowless room in a sturdy building on the lowest level that is not subject to flooding.

- Based on your location and community plans, make your own plans for evacuation or sheltering in place.

- Become familiar with your evacuation zone, the evacuation route, and shelter locations.

- Gather needed supplies for at least three days. Keep in mind each person's specific needs, including medication. Do not forget the needs of pets.

- Keep important documents in a safe place, or create password-protected digital copies.

- Protect your property. Declutter drains and gutters. Install check valves in plumbing to prevent backups. Consider hurricane shutters. Review insurance policies.

When a Hurricane Is 36 Hours from Arriving

- Turn on your TV or radio in order to get the latest weather updates and emergency instructions.

- Restock your emergency preparedness kit. Include food and water sufficient for at least three days, medications, a flashlight, batteries, cash, and first aid supplies.

- Plan how to communicate with family members if you lose power. For example, you can call, text, email, or use social media. Remember that during disasters, sending text messages is usually reliable and faster than making phone calls because phone lines are often overloaded.

- Review your evacuation zone, the evacuation route, and shelter locations. Plan with your family. You may have to leave quickly, so plan ahead.

- Keep your car in good working condition, and keep the gas tank full; stock your vehicle with emergency supplies and a change of clothes.

- If you have the National Flood Insurance Program (NFIP) flood insurance, your policy may cover up to $1,000 in loss avoidance measures, such as sandbags and water pumps, to protect your insured property. You should keep copies of all receipts and a record of the time spent performing the work. They should be submitted to your insurance adjuster when you file a claim to be reimbursed.

When a Hurricane Is 18 to 36 Hours from Arriving

- Bookmark your city or county website for quick access to storm updates and emergency instructions.

- Bring loose, lightweight objects inside that could become projectiles in high winds (e.g., patio furniture, garbage cans); anchor objects that would be unsafe to bring inside (e.g., propane tanks); and trim or remove trees close enough to fall on the building.

- Cover all of your home's windows. Permanent storm shutters offer the best protection for windows. A second option is to board up windows with 5/8" exterior grade or marine plywood, cut to fit and ready to install.

When a Hurricane Is 6 to 18 Hours from Arriving

- Turn on your television (TV)/radio, or check your city/county website every 30 minutes in order to get the latest weather updates and emergency instructions.

- Charge your cell phone now so you will have a fully charged battery if you lose power.

When a Hurricane Is 6 Hours from Arriving

- If you are not in an area that is recommended for evacuation, plan to stay at home or where you are and let friends and family know where you are.

- Close storm shutters, and stay away from windows. Flying glass from broken windows could injure you.

- Turn your refrigerator or freezer to the coldest setting, and open only when necessary. If you lose power, food will last longer. Keep a thermometer in the refrigerator to be able to check the food temperature when the power is restored.

- Turn on your TV/radio, or check your city/county website every 30 minutes in order to get the latest weather updates and emergency instructions.

Survive during a Hurricane

- If told to evacuate, do so immediately. Do not drive around barricades.

- If sheltering during high winds, go to a FEMA safe room, an ICC 500 storm shelter, or a small, interior, windowless room or hallway on the lowest floor that is not subject to flooding.

- If trapped in a building due to flooding, go to the highest level of the building. Do not climb into a closed attic. You may become trapped by rising floodwater.

- Listen for current emergency information and instructions.

- Use a generator or other gasoline-powered machinery outdoors only and away from windows.

- Do not walk, swim, or drive through floodwaters. Turn around; do not drown. Just six inches of fast-moving water can knock you down, and one foot of moving water can sweep your vehicle away.

- Stay off of bridges over fast-moving water.

Be Safe after a Hurricane

- Listen to the authorities for information and special instructions.

- Be careful during cleanup. Wear protective clothing, and work with someone else.

- Do not touch electrical equipment if it is wet or if you are standing in water. If it is safe to do so, turn off electricity at the main breaker or fuse box to prevent electric shock.

- Avoid wading in floodwater, which can contain dangerous debris. Underground or downed power lines can also electrically charge the water.

- Save phone calls for emergencies. Phone systems are often down or busy after a disaster. Use text messages or social media to communicate with family and friends.

- Document any property damage with photographs. Contact your insurance company for assistance.

About Floods

Failing to evacuate flooded areas, entering floodwaters, or remaining after a flood has passed can result in injury or death. Flooding is a temporary overflow of water onto land that is normally dry. Floods are the most common natural disaster in the United States. Floods may:

- Result from rain, snow, coastal storms, storm surges, and overflows of dams and other water systems

- Develop slowly or quickly—flash floods can come with no warning.

- Cause outages, disrupt transportation, damage buildings, and create landslides

If you are under a flood warning, find safe shelter right away.

- Do not walk, swim, or drive through floodwaters. Turn around; do not drown.

  - Just six inches of moving water can knock you down, and one foot of moving water can sweep your vehicle away.

- Stay off of bridges over fast-moving water.

  - Determine how best to protect yourself based on the type of flooding.

  - Evacuate if you are told to do so.

  - Move to higher ground or a higher floor.

- Stay where you are.

How to Stay Safe When a Flood Threatens
Prepare Now for a Flood

- Know types of flood risk in your area. Visit FEMA's Flood Map Service Center for information.

- Sign up for your community's warning system. The EAS and the NOAA Weather Radio also provide emergency alerts.

- If flash flooding is a risk in your location, then monitor potential signs, such as heavy rain.

- Learn and practice evacuation routes, shelter plans, and flash flood response.

- Gather supplies in case you have to leave immediately or if the services are cut off. Keep in mind each person's specific needs, including medication. Do not forget the needs of pets. Obtain extra batteries and charging devices for phones and other critical equipment.

313

- Purchase or renew a flood insurance policy. It typically takes up to 30 days for a policy to go into effect and can protect the life you have built. Homeowner's policies do not cover flooding. Get flood coverage under the National Flood Insurance Program (NFIP).

- Keep important documents in a waterproof container. Create password-protected digital copies.

- Protect your property. Move valuables to higher levels. Declutter drains and gutters. Install check valves. Consider a sump pump with a battery.

Survive during a Flood

- Depending on where you are and the impact and the warning time of flooding, go to the safe location that you previously identified.

- If told to evacuate, do so immediately. Never drive around barricades. Local responders use them to safely direct traffic out of flooded areas.

- Listen to the EAS, the NOAA Weather Radio, or local alerting systems for current emergency information and instructions.

- Do not walk, swim, or drive through floodwaters. Turn around; do not drown.

- Stay off bridges over fast-moving water. Fast-moving water can wash bridges away without warning.

- If your vehicle is trapped in rapidly moving water, then stay inside. If water is rising inside the vehicle, then seek refuge on the roof.

- If trapped in a building, then go to its highest level. Do not climb into a closed attic. You may become trapped by rising floodwater. Go on the roof only if necessary. Once there, signal for help.

Be Safe after a Flood

- Listen to the authorities for information and instructions. Return home only when authorities say it is safe.

- Avoid driving, except in emergencies.

- Snakes and other animals may be in your house. Wear heavy gloves and boots during cleanup.

- Be aware of the risk of electrocution. Do not touch electrical equipment if it is wet or if you are standing in water. If it is safe to do so, turn off the electricity to prevent electric shock.

- Avoid wading in floodwater, which can contain dangerous debris and be contaminated. Underground or downed power lines can also electrically charge the water.

- Use a generator or other gasoline-powered machinery only outdoors and away from windows.

Chapter 57

Thunderstorms and Lightning

Lightning is a leading cause of injury and death from weather-related hazards.

Thunderstorms are dangerous storms that may result in lightning, powerful winds, hail, flash floods, or tornados.

If you are under a thunderstorm warning, find safe shelter right away.

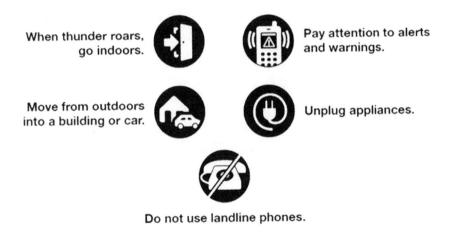

When thunder roars, go indoors.

Pay attention to alerts and warnings.

Move from outdoors into a building or car.

Unplug appliances.

Do not use landline phones.

Figure 57.1. When a Thunderstorm Strikes

About This Chapter: Text in this chapter begins with excerpts from "Be Prepared for a Thunderstorm, Lightning, or Hail," Federal Emergency Management Agency (FEMA), May 2018; Text under the heading "Lightning Myths and Facts" is excerpted from "Lightning Safety Awareness Week," National Weather Service (NWS), June 24, 2012. Reviewed July 2019.

How to Stay Safe When a Thunderstorm Threatens

Prepare Now for Thunderstorm

- Know your area's risk of thunderstorms. They can occur year-round and at any hour.

- Sign up for your community's warning system. The Emergency Alert System (EAS) and the National Oceanic and Atmospheric Administration (NOAA) Weather Radio also provide emergency alerts.

- Identify sturdy buildings close to where you live, work, study, and play.

- Cut down or trim trees that may be in danger of falling on your home.

- Consider buying surge protectors, lightning rods, or a lightning protection system to protect your home, appliances, and electronic devices.

- Secure outside furniture.

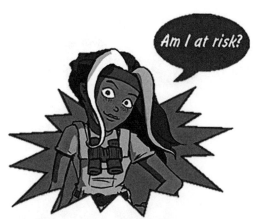

Thunderstorms and lightning happen everywhere, but dry thunderstorms that do not produce rain are most common in the Western United States. They usually occur in the summer when it is warm and humid.

Figure 57.2. Thunderstorms and Lightning: Interesting Fact *(Source: "Thunderstorms and Lightning," Ready, U.S. Department of Homeland Security (DHS).)*

Survive during the Thunderstorm

- **When thunder roars, go indoors.** A sturdy building is the safest place to be during a thunderstorm.

- **Pay attention to weather reports and warnings of thunderstorms.** Be ready to change plans, if necessary, to be near a shelter.

- **When you receive a thunderstorm warning or hear thunder, go inside immediately.**

- **If indoors, avoid running water or using landline phones.** Electricity can travel through plumbing and phone lines.

- **Protect your property.** Unplug appliances and other electronic devices.

- **If boating or swimming,** get to land and find a sturdy, grounded shelter or vehicle immediately.

- **If necessary, take shelter in a car with a metal top and sides.** Do not touch anything metal.

- **Avoid flooded roadways.** Just six inches of fast-moving water can knock you down, and one foot of moving water can sweep your vehicle away.

Be Safe after the Thunderstorm

- **Listen to authorities and weather forecasts** for information on whether it is safe to go outside and instructions regarding potential flash flooding.

- **Watch for fallen power lines and trees.** Report them immediately.

- Take an active role in your safety.

Lightning Myths and Facts

Myth: A lightning victim is electrified. If you touch them, you will risk being electrocuted.

Fact: The human body does not store electricity, and lightning victims require immediate medical attention. It is perfectly safe to touch a lightning victim in order to give them first aid. Call 911 for help.

Myth: If it is not raining or there are no clouds overhead, you are safe from lightning.

Fact: Lightning often strikes several miles from the center of a thunderstorm, far outside the rain or thunderstorm cloud. In fact, "bolts from the blue" can strike as far as 25 miles out from the parent thunderstorm. That is why it is important to seek shelter at the first indication of a thunderstorm and stay there until 30 minutes after the last clap of thunder.

Myth: The rubber soles of shoes or rubber tires on a car will protect you from a lightning strike.

Fact: Rubber-soled shoes and rubber tires provide NO protection from lightning, but most vehicles with metal tops and sides do provide adequate shelter from lightning because the charge travels through the metal frame and eventually into the ground. Just be sure to avoid contact with anything inside the vehicle that conducts electricity. Remember, convertibles, motorcycles, bicycles, open-shelled outdoor recreational vehicles and cars with fiberglass shells offer no protection from lightning.

Myth: "Heat Lightning" occurs after very hot summer days and poses no threat.

Fact: Many people incorrectly think that "heat lightning" is a specific type of lightning. Actually, it is just lightning from a thunderstorm that is too far away for any thunder to be heard (thunder is seldom heard beyond 10 miles under ideal conditions). If the storm approaches, the same lightning safety guidelines above should be followed.

Myth: Lightning never strikes the same place twice.

Fact: Lightning often strikes the same place or object repeatedly, especially if it is tall, pointy, and isolated. The Empire State Building is struck by lightning nearly 100 times each year.

Myth: If caught outside during a thunderstorm, you should seek shelter under a tree.

Fact: Seeking shelter under a tree is one of the leading causes of lightning-related fatalities. Remember, NO PLACE outside is safe when thunderstorms are in the area. If you are caught outside in a thunderstorm, keep moving toward a safe shelter.

Myth: Metal structures or metal on the body (jewelry, watches, etc.) attract lightning.

Fact: The presence of metal has no bearing on where lightning will strike. Mountains are made of rock but get struck by lightning many times a year. Rather, an object's height, shape, and isolation are the dominant factors that affect its likelihood of being struck by lightning. While metal does not attract lightning, it obviously does conduct electricity, so stay away from metal fences, railings, bleachers, etc. during a thunderstorm.

Myth: If caught outside during a thunderstorm, you should lie flat on the ground.

Fact: NO PLACE outside is safe when thunderstorms are in the area. If you are caught outside in a thunderstorm, keep moving toward a safe shelter.

Chapter 58

Be Prepared for Winter Storms

Preparing for a Winter Storm

During extremely cold weather or winter storms, staying warm and safe can be a challenge. Winter storms can bring cold temperatures, power failures, loss of communication services, and icy roads. To keep yourself and your loved ones safe, you should know how to prepare your home and your car before a winter storm hits.

Make a Plan before the Winter Storm

Be prepared before a winter storm hits by planning ahead. If you are in an area prone to winter weather, be sure to create a communication and disaster plan for your family ahead of time.

Prepare Your Home and Car
Weatherproof Your Home

- Insulate any water lines that run along exterior walls, so your water supply will be less likely to freeze.

- Caulk and weather strip doors and windows.

- Insulate walls and attic.

About This Chapter: This chapter includes text excerpted from "Preparing for a Winter Storm," Centers for Disease Control and Prevention (CDC), February 4, 2019.

- Install storm or thermal-pane windows, or cover windows with plastic from the inside.

- Repair roof leaks, and cut away tree branches that could fall on your home or other structure during a storm.

Have Your Chimney or Flue Inspected Each Year

If you plan to use a fireplace or wood stove for emergency heating, have your chimney or flue inspected each year. Ask your local fire department to recommend an inspector, or find one online.

Install a Smoke Detector and a Battery-Operated Carbon Monoxide Detector

- If you will be using a fireplace, wood stove, or kerosene heater, install a smoke detector and a battery-operated carbon monoxide detector near the area to be heated. Test them monthly, and replace batteries twice a year.

- Keep a multipurpose, dry-chemical fire extinguisher nearby.

- All fuel-burning equipment should be vented to the outside.

- Each winter season, have your furnace system and vent checked by a qualified technician to ensure they are functioning properly.

For Older Adults, Keep an Easy-to-Read Thermometer inside Your Home

If a loved one is over 65 years of age, place an easy-to-read thermometer in an indoor location where you will see it frequently. Our ability to feel a change in temperature decreases with age. Older adults are more susceptible to health problems caused by cold. Check the temperature of your home often during the winter months.

Create an Emergency Car Kit

It is best to avoid traveling, but if travel is necessary, keep the following in your car:

- Cell phone, portable charger, and extra batteries

- Items, such as extra hats, coats, mittens, and blankets to keep you warm

- Windshield scraper

- Shovel

- Battery-powered radio with extra batteries

- Flashlight with extra batteries

- Water and snack food

- First aid kit with any necessary medications and a pocket knife

- Tow chains or rope

- Tire chains

- Canned compressed air with sealant for emergency tire repair

- Cat litter or sand to help tires get traction, or road salt to melt ice

- Booster cables with a fully charged battery or jumper cables

- Hazard or other reflectors

- Bright colored flag or help signs, emergency distress flag, and/or emergency flares

- Road maps

- Waterproof matches and a can to melt snow for water

Steps to Take before the Storm Hits
Listen to Weather Forecasts and Check Your Supplies

Listen to weather forecasts regularly, and check your emergency supplies, including your emergency food and water supply, whenever you are expecting a winter storm or extreme cold. Even though we cannot always predict extreme cold in advance, weather forecasts can sometimes give you several days of notice to prepare.

Bring Your Pets Indoors

If you have pets, bring them indoors. If you cannot bring them inside, provide adequate shelter to keep them warm and make sure they have access to unfrozen water.

Get Your Car Ready

Have maintenance service on your vehicle as often as the manufacturer recommends. In addition, every fall, do the following:

- Have the radiator system serviced, or check the antifreeze level yourself with an antifreeze tester. Add antifreeze as needed.

- Replace windshield-wiper fluid with a wintertime mixture.

- Make sure the tires on your car have adequate tread and air pressure. Replace any worn tires, and fill low tires with air to the proper pressure recommended for your car (typically between 30 to 35 psi).

- Keep the gas tank near full to help avoid ice in the tank and fuel lines.

- Keep your car in good working order. Be sure to check the following: heater, defroster, brakes, brake fluid, ignition, emergency flashers, exhaust, oil, and battery.

Stay Safe during and after a Winter Storm

Winter storms are dangerous. They can bring cold temperatures, power failures, loss of communication services, and icy roads. This can make being outside dangerous, so you should limit your time outside. Although staying indoors as much as possible can help reduce the risk of car crashes and falls on the ice, you may also face hazards inside your home.

Stay Safe Indoors

Protect yourself and your loved ones during a winter storm. Take extra steps to make sure your home is heated safely, and follow the tips below.

Heat Your Home Safely

If you plan to use a wood stove, fireplace, or space heater, be extremely careful. Follow the manufacturer's instructions, and remember these safety tips:

- Turning on the stove for heat is not safe; have at least one of the following heat sources in case the power goes out:

  - Extra blankets, sleeping bags, and warm winter coats

  - Fireplace that is up to code with plenty of dry firewood or a gas log fireplace

  - Portable space heaters or kerosene heaters. Check with your local fire department to make sure that kerosene heaters are legal in your area.

- Use electric space heaters with automatic shut-off switches and nonglowing elements. Make sure to keep them away from any flammable materials, such as curtains or blankets.

- Use fireplaces, wood stoves, or other combustion heaters only if they are properly vented to the outside and do not leak gas from the flue or exhaust into the indoor air space.

- Have your heating system serviced by a qualified technician every year.

- Do not burn paper in a fireplace.

- Make sure you have proper ventilation if you must use a kerosene heater.

- Use only the type of fuel your heater is designed to use—do not substitute.

- Keep heat sources, such as space heaters, at least three feet away from drapes, furniture, or bedding. Never cover your space heater.

- Never place a space heater on top of furniture or near water.

- Never leave children unattended near a space heater.

- Make sure that the cord of an electric space heater is not a tripping hazard, but do not run the cord under carpets or rugs.

- Avoid using extension cords to plug in your space heater.

- If your space heater has a damaged electrical cord or produces sparks, do not use it.

Light Your Home Safely

If there is a power failure:

- Use battery-powered flashlights or lanterns rather than candles, if possible. Candles can lead to house fires.

  - If you do use candles, never leave lit candles unattended.

Use Generators and Other Appliances Safely

- Generators should be located at least 20 feet from any window, door, or vent and in a space where rain and snow will not reach them.

- Protect yourself from carbon monoxide (CO) poisoning by installing a battery-operated CO detector.

- Never use generators, gas or charcoal grills, camp stoves, or similar devices inside your home, in basements, in garages, or near windows. The fumes are deadly.

- Plug in appliances to the generator using individual heavy-duty, outdoor-rated extension cords.

- Do not use the generator or appliances if they are wet.

- Do not store gasoline indoors where the fumes could ignite.

Conserve Heat

- Some gas-fueled heaters, such as ventless gas fireplaces, require some ventilation. Otherwise, if you do not need extra ventilation, keep as much heat as possible inside your home.

- Avoid unnecessarily opening doors or windows.

- Close off unneeded rooms.

- Stuff towels or rags in cracks under doors.

- Close draperies or cover windows with blankets at night.

Make Sure Babies and Older Adults Stay Warm

Babies. Infants less than one year of age should never sleep in a cold room because they lose body heat more easily than adults. Follow these tips to keep a baby safe and warm during the extreme cold:

- Remove any pillows or other soft bedding. These can increase the risk of smothering and sudden infant death syndrome (SIDS).

- Dress babies in warmer clothing, such as footed pajamas, one-piece wearable blankets, or sleep sacks.

- Try to maintain a warm temperature inside your home. If you are not able to keep your home warm, make temporary arrangements to stay elsewhere.

- In an emergency, you can keep a baby warm using your own body heat. If you must sleep, take precautions to prevent rolling on or smothering the baby.

Older adults. Older adults often make less body heat because of a slower metabolism and less physical activity. Check on elderly friends and neighbors often to make sure that their homes are heated properly. If anyone in your home is over 65 years of age, check the temperature in your home often during extremely cold weather.

Keep a Water Supply

Extreme cold can cause water pipes in your home to freeze and sometimes rupture, or break. When you are expecting very cold or freezing temperatures:

- Leave all water taps slightly open so they drip continuously.
- Keep the temperature inside your home warm.
- Allow heated air to reach pipes. For example, open cabinet doors beneath the kitchen and bathroom sinks.
- If your pipes do freeze, do not thaw them with a torch. Thaw the pipes slowly with warm air from an electric hair dryer.
- If you cannot thaw your pipes, or the pipes have broken open, use bottled water or get water from a neighbor's home.
- As an emergency measure, if no other water is available, snow can be melted for water. Bringing water to a rolling boil for one minute will kill most germs but will not get rid of chemicals sometimes found in snow.

Eat Well-Balanced Meals and Avoid Alcoholic or Caffeinated Drinks

Eating well-balanced meals will help you stay warmer. Do not drink alcoholic or caffeinated beverages—they cause your body to lose heat faster. Instead, drink warm, sweet beverages or broth to help keep yourself warm. If you have any dietary restrictions, ask your doctor.

Stay Safe Outdoors

Try to stay indoors during extremely cold weather. Make any trips outside as brief as possible, and remember the tips below to protect your health and safety.

Dress Warmly and Stay Dry

Adults and children should wear:

- A hat
- A scarf or knit mask to cover the face and mouth
- Sleeves that are snug at the wrist
- Mittens (they are warmer than gloves)

- Water-resistant coat and boots

- Several layers of loose-fitting clothing

Layer-Up

- **Inner layer:** Wear fabrics that will hold more body heat and do not absorb moisture. Wool, silk, or polypropylene will hold more body heat than cotton.

- **Insulation layer:** An insulation layer will help you retain heat by trapping air close to your body. Natural fibers, such as wool, goose down, or a fleece, work best.

- **Outer layer:** The outermost layer helps protect you from wind, rain, and snow. It should be tightly woven and preferably water and wind resistant to reduce the loss of body heat.

Additional tips:

- Stay dry—wet clothing chills the body quickly.

- Excess sweating will cause your body to lose more heat, so remove extra layers of clothing whenever you feel too warm.

- Avoid getting gasoline or alcohol on your skin while de-icing and fueling your car or using a snow blower. Getting these materials on your skin will cause your body to lose a lot more heat.

- Do not ignore shivering—it is an important first sign that your body is losing heat. Constant shivering is a sign that it is time to go inside.

Know the Signs of Frostbite and Hypothermia

Hypothermia (abnormally low body temperature) is a dangerous condition that can happen when a person is exposed to extremely cold temperatures.

In adults, warning signs of hypothermia include shivering, exhaustion or feeling very tired, confusion, fumbling hands, memory loss, slurred speech, and drowsiness. In babies, signs include bright red, cold skin and very low energy.

If you notice any of these signs, take the person's temperature. If it is below 95 °F, the situation is an emergency—get medical attention immediately.

Frostbite is a type of injury caused by freezing. It can lead to a loss of feeling and color in the areas it affects, usually the nose, ears, cheeks, chin, fingers, and toes. Frostbite can permanently damage the body, and severe cases can lead to amputation (removing the affected body part).

Signs of frostbite include a white or grayish-yellow skin area, skin that feels unusually firm or waxy, and numbness. If you notice signs of frostbite, seek medical care.

Stay off the ice. Walking on ice is extremely dangerous. Many injuries related to cold weather happen from falls on ice-covered sidewalks, steps, driveways, and porches. Keep your steps and walkways as free of ice as possible by using rock salt or another chemical de-icing compound. Sand may also be used on walkways to reduce the risk of slipping.

What to Expect during Cleanup

Cold weather puts an extra strain on the heart. If you have heart disease or high blood pressure, follow your doctor's advice about shoveling snow or performing other hard work in the cold. Otherwise, if you have to do heavy outdoor chores, dress warmly and work slowly to avoid excess sweating. Remember, your body is already working hard just to stay warm, so do not overdo it.

Be Safe during Outdoor Activities

- Let your friends and family know where you will be before you go hiking, camping, or skiing.

- Do not leave any areas of your skin exposed to the cold.

- Try not to sweat or become too tired.

- Be prepared to take emergency shelter.

- Pack dry clothing, a two-way radio, waterproof matches, and paraffin fire starters with you.

- Do not use alcohol and other mood-altering substances, and avoid caffeinated drinks.

- Avoid walking on ice or getting wet.

- Carefully watch for signs of cold-weather health problems, such as hypothermia and frostbite.

Be Careful While Traveling

- Listen for radio or television reports of travel advisories issued by the National Weather Service (NWS).

- Do not travel in low visibility conditions.

- Avoid traveling on ice-covered roads, overpasses, and bridges if at all possible.

- Never pour water on your windshield to remove ice or snow—this can cause your windshield to shatter.

- If you must travel by car, use tire chains and take a mobile phone with you.

- If you must travel, let someone know your destination and when you expect to arrive. Ask them to notify the authorities if you are late.

- Check and restock the winter emergency supplies in your car before you leave.

- Always carry extra warm clothing and blankets with you. Do not rely on a car to provide enough heat. The car could break down.

If You Get Stranded in Your Car

Staying in your car when you are stranded is often the safest choice if winter storms create poor visibility or if roadways are ice covered. These steps will increase your safety when stranded:

- Tie a brightly colored cloth to the antenna as a signal to rescuers, and raise the hood of the car (if it is not snowing).

- Move anything you need from the trunk into the passenger area.

- Wrap your entire body, including your head, in extra clothing, blankets, or newspapers.

- Stay awake. You will be less vulnerable to cold-related health problems.

- Run the motor (and heater) for about 10 minutes per hour, opening 1 window slightly to let in air. Make sure that snow is not blocking the exhaust pipe—this will reduce the risk of CO poisoning.

- As you sit, keep moving your arms and legs to improve your circulation and stay warmer.

- Do not eat snow because it will lower your body temperature.

- Huddle with other people for warmth.

Prevent Hypothermia and Frostbite

Hypothermia and frostbite are both dangerous conditions that can happen when a person is exposed to extremely cold temperatures. Stay safe this winter by learning more about hypothermia and frostbite, including who is most at risk, signs, and symptoms, and what to do if someone develops hypothermia or frostbite.

Hypothermia

What Is Hypothermia?

Hypothermia is caused by prolonged exposure to very cold temperatures. When exposed to cold temperatures, your body begins to lose heat faster than it is produced. Lengthy exposures will eventually use up your body's stored energy, which leads to lower body temperature.

Body temperature that is too low affects the brain, making the victim unable to think clearly or move well. This makes hypothermia dangerous because a person may not know that it is happening and will not be able to do anything about it.

While hypothermia is most likely at very cold temperatures, it can occur even at cool temperatures (above 40°F) if a person becomes chilled from rain, sweat, or submersion in cold water.

Who Is Most at Risk?

Victims of hypothermia are often:

- Older adults with inadequate food, clothing, or heating
- Babies sleeping in cold bedrooms
- People who remain outdoors for long periods—the homeless, hikers, hunters, etc.
- People who drink alcohol or use illicit drugs

What Are the Signs and Symptoms of Hypothermia?

The following are warning signs of hypothermia:

Adults:

- Shivering
- Exhaustion or feeling very tired
- Confusion
- Fumbling hands
- Memory loss
- Slurred speech
- Drowsiness

Babies:

- Bright red, cold skin

- Very low energy

Do Not Wait—Take Action

Hypothermia is a medical emergency. If you notice any of the above signs, take the person's temperature. If it is below 95 °F, get medical attention immediately.

If you are not able to get medical help right away, try to warm the person up.

- Get the person into a warm room or shelter.

- Remove any wet clothing the person is wearing.

- Warm the center of the person's body—chest, neck, head, and groin—using an electric blanket, if available. You can also use skin-to-skin contact under loose, dry layers of blankets, clothing, towels, or sheets.

- Warm drinks can help increase body temperature, but do not give the person alcoholic drinks. Do not try to give beverages to an unconscious person.

- After body temperature has increased, keep the person dry and wrap their body, including their head and neck, in a warm blanket.

- Get the person proper medical attention as soon as possible.

A person with severe hypothermia may be unconscious and may not seem to have a pulse or to be breathing. In this case, handle the person gently, and get emergency assistance immediately.

- Perform cardiopulmonary resuscitation (CPR), even if the person appears dead. CPR should continue until the person responds or medical aid becomes available. Keep warming the person while performing CPR. In some cases, hypothermia victims who appear to be dead can be successfully resuscitated.

Frostbite
What Is Frostbite?

Frostbite is a type of injury caused by freezing. It leads to a loss of feeling and color in the areas it affects, usually extremities, such as the nose, ears, cheeks, chin, fingers, and toes. Frostbite can permanently damage the body, and severe cases can lead to amputation.

Who Is Most at Risk?

You may have a greater chance of developing frostbite if you

- Have poor blood circulation

- Are not properly dressed for extremely cold temperatures

What Are the Signs and Symptoms of Frostbite?

If you notice redness or pain in any skin area, get out of the cold or protect any exposed skin—frostbite may be beginning. Any of the following signs may point to frostbite:

- A white or grayish-yellow skin area

- Skin that feels unusually firm or waxy

- Numbness

- A person who has frostbite may not know they have it until someone else points it out because the frozen parts of their body are numb.

Do Not Wait—Take Action!

If you notice signs of frostbite on yourself or someone else, seek medical care. Check to see if the person is also showing signs of hypothermia. Hypothermia is a more serious condition and requires emergency medical care.

If a person shows signs of frostbite but no signs of hypothermia and immediate medical care is not available, do the following:

- Get the person into a warm room as soon as possible.

- Unless absolutely necessary, do not walk on feet or toes that show signs of frostbite—this increases the damage.

- Do not rub the frostbitten area with snow or massage it at all. This can cause more damage.

- Put the areas affected by frostbite in warm—not hot—water (the temperature should be comfortable to the touch for unaffected parts of the body).

- If warm water is not available, warm the affected area using body heat. For example, you can use the heat of an armpit to warm frostbitten fingers.

- Do not use a heating pad; heat lamp; or the heat of a stove, fireplace, or radiator for warming. Affected areas are numb and can easily burn.

Do not substitute these steps for proper medical care. Frostbite should be checked by a healthcare provider. And remember, hypothermia is a medical emergency, and immediate medical care is necessary.

Be Prepared

Taking a first aid or emergency resuscitation course is a good way to prepare for health problems related to cold weather. Knowing what to do is an important part of protecting your health and the health of others.

Being prepared is your best defense against having to deal with extremely cold weather. By preparing your home and car ahead of winter storms or other winter emergencies, and by taking safety precautions during extremely cold weather, you can reduce your risk of developing health problems related to cold weather.

Chapter 59

Chemical Emergencies

Chemical agents are poisonous vapors, aerosols, liquids, and solids that have toxic effects on people, animals, or plants. While potentially lethal, chemical agents are difficult to deliver in lethal concentrations because they dissipate rapidly outdoors and are difficult to produce.

Before a Chemical Emergency

A chemical attack could come without warning. Signs of a chemical release include people having difficulty breathing; eye irritation; loss of coordination; nausea; or burning in the nose, throat, and lungs. The presence of many dead insects or birds may indicate a chemical agent release.

What you should do to prepare for a chemical threat:

- Build an emergency supply kit and include:

  - Duct tape

  - Scissors

  - Plastic to cover doors, windows, and vents

- Make a family emergency plan.

About This Chapter: This chapter includes text excerpted from "Chemical Emergencies," Ready, U.S. Department of Homeland Security (DHS), July 31, 2017.

During a Chemical Emergency

What you should do in a chemical attack:

- Quickly try to define the impacted area or where the chemical is coming from, if possible.

- Take immediate action to get away.

- If the chemical is inside a building where you are, get out of the building without passing through the contaminated area, if possible.

- If you cannot get out of the building or find clean air without passing through the affected area, move as far away as possible and shelter in place.

If you are instructed to remain in your home or office building, you should:

- Close the doors and windows, and turn off all ventilation, including furnaces, air conditioners, vents, and fans.

- Seek shelter in an internal room with your disaster supplies kit.

- Seal the room with duct tape and plastic sheeting.

- Listen to the radio or television for instructions from the authorities.

If you are caught in or near a contaminated area outdoors:

- Quickly decide what is the fastest way to find clean air:

    - Move away immediately and in a direction upwind of the source.

    - Find the closest building to shelter in place.

After a Chemical Emergency

Do not leave the safety of a shelter to go outdoors to help others until the authorities announce that it is safe to do so.

A person affected by a chemical agent requires immediate medical attention from a professional. If medical help is not immediately available, decontaminate yourself and assist in decontaminating others.

Decontamination guidelines are as follows:

- Use extreme caution when helping others who have been exposed to chemical agents.

- Remove all clothing and other items in contact with the body.

- Cut off clothing normally removed over the head to avoid contact with the eyes, nose, and mouth.

- Put contaminated clothing and items into a plastic bag and seal it.

- Remove eyeglasses or contact lenses. Put glasses in a pan of household bleach to decontaminate them and then rinse and dry.

- Wash hands with soap and water.

- Flush eyes with water.

- Gently wash face and hair with soap and water before thoroughly rinsing with water.

- Proceed to a medical facility for screening and professional treatment.

Chapter 60

National Security Emergencies

National Terrorism Advisory System

The U.S. Department of Homeland Security's (DHS) National Terrorism Advisory System (NTAS) informs the public and relevant government and private sector partners about potential or actual threats, indicating whether there is an "imminent" or "elevated" threat.

Report suspicious activity to local law enforcement, or call 911.

What to Do If There Is a Bomb Threat

Bomb threats or suspicious items should always be taken seriously. How quickly and safely you react to a bomb threat could save lives, including your own.

If You Receive a Bomb Threat

Bomb threats are most commonly received via phone, but they are also made in person, via an email, a written note, or other means. Every bomb threat is unique and should be handled in the context of the facility or environment in which it occurs. Facility supervisors and law

About This Chapter: Text under the heading "National Terrorism Advisory System" is excerpted from "DHS National Terrorism Advisory System," U.S. General Services Administration (GSA), February 26, 2019; Text under the heading "What to Do If There Is a Bomb Threat" is excerpted from "What to Do—Bomb Threat," U.S. Department of Homeland Security (DHS), August 22, 2018; Text under the heading "What to Do if There Is a Nuclear Explosion" is excerpted from "Nuclear Explosion," Ready, Department of Homeland Security (DHS), February 10, 2018.

enforcement will be in the best position to determine the credibility of the threat. Follow these procedures:

- Remain calm.

- Notify the authorities immediately:

  - Notify your facility supervisors, such as a manager, operator, or administrator, or follow your facility's standard operating procedure.

  - Call 911 or your local law enforcement if no facility supervisor is available.

- For threats made via phone:

  - Keep the caller on the line as long as possible. Be polite, and show interest to keep them talking.

  - Do not hang up, even if the caller does.

  - If possible, signal or pass a note to other staff members to listen and to help notify the authorities.

  - Write down as much information as possible—caller ID number, exact wording of threat, type of voice or behavior, etc.—that will aid investigators.

  - Record the call, if possible.

- Be available for interviews with facility supervisors and/or law enforcement.

- Follow the authorities' instructions. Facility supervisors and/or law enforcement will assess the situation and provide guidance regarding facility lockdown, search, and/or evacuation

If You Find a Suspicious Item

Together we can help keep our communities safe—if you see something that is suspicious, out of place, or does not look right, say something. A suspicious item is any item (e.g., bag, package, vehicle, etc.) that is reasonably believed to contain explosives, an improvised explosive device (IED), or other hazardous material that requires a bomb technician and/or specialized equipment to further evaluate it. Examples that could indicate a bomb include unexplainable wires or electronics; other visible bomb-like components; and unusual sounds, vapors, mists, or odors. Generally speaking, anything that is Hidden, Obviously suspicious, and not Typical (HOT) should be deemed suspicious. In addition, potential indicators for a bomb are threats, placement, and proximity of the item to people and valuable assets.

You may encounter a suspicious item unexpectedly. If it appears to be a suspicious item, follow these procedures:

- Remain calm.

- Do not touch, tamper with, or move the package, bag, or item.

- Notify the authorities immediately:

  - Notify your facility supervisors, such as a manager, operator, or administrator, or follow your facility's standard operating procedure.

  - Call 911 or your local law enforcement if no facility supervisor is available.

  - Explain why it appears suspicious.

- Follow instructions. Facility supervisors and/or law enforcement will assess the situation and provide guidance regarding shelter in place or evacuation.

- If no guidance is provided and you feel you are in immediate danger, calmly evacuate the area. Distance and protective cover are the best ways to reduce injury from a bomb.

- Be aware. There could be other threats or suspicious items.

Every situation is unique and should be handled in the context of the facility or environment in which it occurs. Facility supervisors and law enforcement will be in the best position to determine if a real risk is posed and how to respond.

> **Note: Not all items are suspicious.** An unattended item is an item (e.g., bag, package, vehicle, etc.) of unknown origin and content where there are no obvious signs of being suspicious. Facility search, lock-down, or evacuation is not necessary unless the item is determined to be suspicious.

To report suspicious activity, call 911 or contact local law enforcement.

Please contact your local Protective Security Advisor (PSA) or send an email to the Office for Bombing Prevention (OBP) at OBP@hq.dhs.gov for additional information about OBP products and programs or to schedule a training session or a planning workshop.

Informed, alert communities play a critical role in keeping our nation safe. Everyone has a responsibility to protect our nation.

What to Do if There Is a Nuclear Explosion

Nuclear explosions can cause significant damage and casualties from blast, heat, and radiation, but you can keep your family safe by knowing what to do and being prepared if it occurs.

A nuclear weapon is a device that uses a nuclear reaction to create an explosion. Nuclear devices range from a small portable device carried by an individual to a weapon carried by a missile. A nuclear explosion may occur with or without a few minutes warning.

Fallout is most dangerous in the first few hours after the detonation when it is giving off the highest levels of radiation. It takes time for the fallout to arrive back to ground level, often more than 15 minutes for areas outside of the immediate blast damage zones. This is enough time for you to be able to prevent significant radiation exposure by following these simple steps:

Get inside. Get inside the nearest building to avoid radiation. Brick or concrete buildings are best.

- Remove contaminated clothing, and wipe off or wash unprotected skin if you were outside after the fallout arrived.

- Go to the basement or middle of the building. Stay away from the outer walls and roof.

Stay inside. Stay inside for 24 hours unless local authorities provide other instructions.

- Other family members should stay where they are inside. Reunite later to avoid exposure to dangerous radiation.

- Keep your pets inside.

Stay tuned. Tune into any media available for official information, such as when it is safe to exit and where you should go.

- Battery operated and hand crank radios will function after a nuclear detonation.

- Cell phone, text messaging, television, and Internet services may be disrupted or unavailable.

How to Stay Safe in the Event of a Nuclear Explosion
Prepare Now for a Nuclear Explosion

Identify shelter locations. Identify the best shelter location near where you spend a lot of time, such as home, work, and school. The best locations are underground and in the middle of larger buildings.

While commuting, identify appropriate shelters to seek in the event of a detonation.

Outdoor areas, vehicles, mobile homes do not provide adequate shelter. Look for basements or the center of large multistory buildings.

Make sure you have an emergency supply kit for places you frequent and might have to stay at for 24 hours. It should include bottled water, packaged foods, emergency medicines, a hand-crank or battery-powered radio to get information in case the power is out, a flashlight, and extra batteries for essential items. If possible, store supplies for three or more days.

Survive during a Nuclear Explosion

If warned of an imminent attack, immediately get inside the nearest building and move away from windows. This will help provide protection from the blast, heat, and radiation of the detonation.

If you are outdoors when a detonation occurs, take cover from the blast behind anything that might offer protection. Lie face down to protect exposed skin from the heat and flying debris. If you are in a vehicle, stop safely, and duck down within the vehicle.

After the shock wave passes, get inside the nearest, best shelter location for protection from potential fallout. You will have 10 minutes or more to find adequate shelter.

Be inside before the fallout arrives. The highest outdoor radiation levels from fallout occur immediately after the fallout arrives and then decrease with time.

Stay tuned for updated instructions from emergency response officials. If advised to evacuate, listen for information about routes, shelters, and procedures.

If you have evacuated, do not return until you are told it is safe to do so by local officials.

Be Safe after a Nuclear Explosion

Immediately after you are inside shelter, if you may have been outside after the fallout arrived:

- Remove your outer layer of contaminated clothing to remove fallout and radiation from your body.
- Take a shower or wash with soap and water to remove fallout from any skin or hair that was not covered. If you cannot wash or shower, use a wipe or clean wet cloth to wipe any skin or hair that was not covered.
- Clean any pets that were outside after the fallout arrived. Gently brush your pet's coat to remove any fallout particles, and wash your pet with soap and water, if available.

- It is safe to eat or drink packaged food items or items that were inside a building. Do not consume food or liquids that were outdoors uncovered and may be contaminated by fallout.

- If you are sick or injured, listen for instructions on how and where to get medical attention when authorities tell you it is safe to exit.

Hazards Related to Nuclear Explosions

- The bright flash can cause temporary blindness for less than a minute.

- A blast wave can cause death, injury, and damage to structures several miles out from the blast.

- Radiation can damage the cells of the body. Large exposures can cause radiation sickness.

- Fire and heat can cause death, burn injuries, and damage to structures several miles out.

- An electromagnetic pulse (EMP) can damage electrical power equipment and electronics several miles out from the detonation and cause temporary disruptions further out.

- Fallout is radioactive, visible dirt and debris raining down from several miles up that can cause sickness to those who are outside.

Chapter 61

Terrorism: Preparing for the Unexpected

Protecting the United States from terrorist attacks is the Federal Bureau of Investigation's (FBI) number one priority. The Bureau employs a variety of disciplines and works closely with a range of partners to neutralize terrorist cells and operatives in the U.S., to help dismantle extremist networks worldwide, and to cut off financing and other forms of support provided to foreign terrorist organizations by terrorist sympathizers. In particular, the FBI-led Joint Terrorism Task Forces (JTTFs) across the country are essential to the nation's success in combatting terrorism. These JTTFs bring federal, state, and local agencies together on one team, allowing members to leverage one another's skills, authorities, and accesses to prevent and disrupt terrorist attacks across the country. The JTTFs also build relationships between the community and law enforcement on the front line, which is particularly important to combatting terrorism.

Terrorism Definitions

International terrorism: Perpetrated by individuals and/or groups inspired by or associated with designated foreign terrorist organizations or nations (state-sponsored). For example, the December 2, 2015 shooting in San Bernardino, CA, that killed 14 people and wounded 22, which involved a married couple who radicalized for some time prior to the attack and were inspired by multiple extremist ideologies and foreign terrorist organizations.

Domestic terrorism: Perpetrated by individuals and/or groups inspired by or associated with primarily U.S.-based movements that espouse extremist ideologies of a political, religious,

About This Chapter: This chapter includes text excerpted from "Terrorism," Federal Bureau of Investigation (FBI), October 24, 2017.

social, racial, or environmental nature. For example, the June 8, 2014, Las Vegas shooting, during which two police officers inside a restaurant were killed in an ambush-style attack, which was committed by a married couple who held anti-government views and who intended to use the shooting to start a revolution.

The Current Threat

The FBI is committed to remaining agile in its approach to terrorism threat, which has continued to evolve significantly since September 11, 2001, terror attacks on the U.S. soil. The threat landscape has expanded considerably, though it is important to note that the more traditional threat posed by al Qaeda and its affiliates is still present and active. The threat of domestic terrorism also remains persistent overall, with actors crossing the line from the first amendment protected rights to committing crimes to further their political agenda.

Three factors have contributed to the evolution of the terrorism threat landscape:

- **The Internet:** International and domestic actors have developed an extensive presence on the Internet through messaging platforms and online images, videos, and publications, which facilitate the groups' ability to radicalize and recruit individuals receptive to extremist messaging. Such messaging is constantly available to people participating in social networks dedicated to various causes, particularly younger people comfortable with communicating in the social media environment.

- **Use of social media:** In addition to using the Internet, social media has allowed both international and domestic terrorists to gain unprecedented, virtual access to people living in the United States in an effort to enable homeland attacks. ISIS, in particular, encourages sympathizers to carry out simple attacks where they are located against targets—in particular, soft targets—or to travel to ISIS-held territory in Iraq and Syria and join its ranks as foreign fighters. This message has resonated with supporters in the United States and abroad, and several attackers have claimed to be acting on ISIS' behalf.

- **Homegrown violent extremists (HVEs):** The FBI, however, cannot focus solely on the terrorist threat emanating from overseas—we also must identify those sympathizers who have radicalized and become HVEs within the United States and aspire to attack the nation from within. HVEs are defined by the Bureau as "global-jihad-inspired individuals who are based in the U.S., have been radicalized primarily in the U.S., and are not directly collaborating with a foreign terrorist organization." The FBI investigates suspected HVEs in every state.

How Citizens Can Protect Themselves and Report Suspicious Activity

It is important for people to protect themselves both online and in person, and to report any suspicious activity they encounter. The simplest way to accomplish this is to:

- Remain aware of your surroundings.

- Refrain from oversharing personal information.

- Say something if you see something.

Nationwide Suspicious Activity Reporting Initiative

The Nationwide Suspicious Activity Reporting (SAR) Initiative is a joint collaborative effort by the U.S. Department of Homeland Security (DHS); the FBI; and state, local, tribal, and territorial law enforcement partners. This initiative provides law enforcement with another tool to help prevent terrorism and other related criminal activity by establishing a national capacity for gathering, documenting, processing, analyzing, and sharing SAR information.

Community Preparedness Tools

Businesses are encouraged to connect, plan, train, and report. Applying these four steps prior to an incident or attack can help better prepare businesses and their employees to proactively think about the role they play in the safety and security of their businesses and communities.

Chapter 62

Bioterrorism

Biological agents are organisms or toxins that can kill or incapacitate people, livestock, and crops. A biological attack is the deliberate release of germs or other biological substances that can make you sick.

There are three basic groups of biological agents that could likely be used as weapons: bacteria, viruses, and toxins. Biological agents can be dispersed by spraying them into the air, person-to-person contact, infecting animals that carry the disease to humans, and by contaminating food and water.

> Biological agents spread through the air, water, or in food. Some can also spread from person to person. They can be very hard to detect. They do not cause illness for several hours or days. Scientists worry that anthrax, botulism, Ebola, and other hemorrhagic fever viruses, plague, or smallpox could be used as biological agents.
>
> *(Source: "Biodefense and Bioterrorism," MedlinePlus.gov, National Institutes of Health (NIH).)*

Before a Biological Threat

A biological attack may or may not be immediately obvious. In most cases, local healthcare workers will report a pattern of unusual illness or there will be a wave of sick people seeking emergency medical attention. The public would be alerted through an emergency radio or TV

About This Chapter: This chapter includes text excerpted from "Bioterrorism," Ready, U.S. Department of Homeland Security (DHS), July 31, 2017.

broadcast, or some other signal used in your community, such as a telephone call or a home visit from an emergency response worker.

> Biodefense uses medical measures to protect people against bioterrorism. This includes medicines and vaccinations. It also includes medical research and preparations to defend against bioterrorist attacks.
>
> *(Source: "Biodefense and Bioterrorism," MedlinePlus.gov, National Institutes of Health (NIH).)*

To protect yourself, your family, and your property from the effects of a biological threat you should build an emergency supply kit.

Make a family emergency plan. Check with your doctor to ensure all required or suggested immunizations are up to date for yourself, your children, and elderly family members.

Consider installing a High-Efficiency Particulate Air (HEPA) filter in your furnace return duct, which will filter out most biological agents that may enter your house.

During a Biological Threat

The first evidence of an attack may be when you notice symptoms of the disease caused by exposure to an agent. In the event of a biological attack, public-health officials may not immediately be able to provide information on what you should do. It will take time to determine exactly what the illness is, how it should be treated, and who is in danger.

Follow these guidelines during a biological threat:

- Watch TV, listen to the radio, or check the Internet for official news and information, including signs and symptoms of the disease, areas in danger, if medications or vaccinations are being distributed, and where you should seek medical attention if you become ill.

- If you become aware of an unusual and suspicious substance, quickly get away.

- Cover your mouth and nose with layers of fabric that can filter the air but still allow breathing. Examples include two to three layers of cotton such as a T-shirt, handkerchief, or towel.

- Depending on the situation, wear a face mask to reduce inhaling or spreading germs.

- If you have been exposed to a biological agent, remove and bag your clothes and personal items. Follow official instructions for disposal of contaminated items.

- Wash yourself with soap and water and put on clean clothes.

- Contact authorities and seek medical assistance. You may be advised to stay away from others or even quarantined.

- If your symptoms match those described and you are in the group considered at risk, immediately seek emergency medical attention.

- Follow instructions of doctors and other public-health officials.

- If the disease is contagious, expect to receive medical evaluation and treatment.

- For noncontagious diseases, expect to receive medical evaluation and treatment.

- In a declared biological emergency or developing epidemic avoid crowds.

- Wash your hands with soap and water frequently.

- Do not share food or utensils.

After a Biological Threat

Pay close attention to all official warnings and instructions on how to proceed. The delivery of medical services for a biological event may be handled differently to respond to increased demand.

The basic public-health procedures and medical protocols for handling exposure to biological agents are the same as for any infectious disease. It is important for you to pay attention to official instructions via radio, television, and emergency-alert systems.

Part Seven
If You Need More Information

Chapter 63

Resources for Information about First Aid and Medical Emergencies

American Academy of Neurology (AAN)

201 Chicago Ave.
Minneapolis, MN 55415
Toll-Free: 800-879-1960
Phone: 612-928-6000
Fax: 612-454-2746
Website: www.aan.com
E-mail: memberservices@aan.com

American Association of Poison Control Centers (AAPCC)

515 King St.
Ste. 510
Alexandria, VA 22314
Toll-Free: 800-222-1222
Website: www.aapcc.org

American Burn Association (ABA)

311 S. Wacker Dr.
Ste. 4150
Chicago, IL 60606-6671
Phone: 312-642-9260
Website: www.ameriburn.org

About This Chapter: Resources in this chapter were compiled from several sources deemed reliable; all contact information was verified and updated in July 2019.

American College of Emergency Physicians (ACEP)

4950 W. Royal Ln.
P.O. Box 619911
Irving, TX 75063-2524
Toll-Free: 800-798-1822
Phone: 972-550-0911
Fax: 972-580-2816
Website: www.acep.org

American Public Health Association Injury Control and Emergency Services (APHA)

800 First St. N.W.
Washington, DC 20001
Phone: 202-777-APHA (202-777-2742)
TTY: 202-777-2500
Fax: 202-777-2534
Website: www.apha.org

American Red Cross

National Headquarters
431 18th St. N.W.
Washington, DC 20006
Toll-Free: 800-RED-CROSS (800-733-2767)
Phone: 202-303-4498
Website: www.redcross.org

American Trauma Society (ATS)

201 Park Washington Ct.
Falls Church, VA 22046
Toll-Free: 800-556-7890
Phone: 703-538-3544
Fax: 703-241-5603
Website: www.amtrauma.org
E-mail: info@amtrauma.org

Brain Injury Association of America (BIAA)
1608 Spring Hill Rd.
Ste. 110
Vienna, VA 22182
Phone: 703-761-0750
Fax: 703-761-0755
Website: www.biausa.org
E-mail: info@biausa.org

Burn and Shock Trauma Research Institute (BSTRI)
Loyola University Chicago
2160 South First Ave.
CTRE Bldg. 115 Rm. 315
Maywood, IL 60153
Website: www.ssom.luc.edu
E-mail: BSTI@luc.edu

Emergency Medical Services for Children (EMSC)
5901 Lincoln Dr.
CBC-ADV-3
Edina, MN 55436
Toll-Free: 800-660-7022
Phone: 612-813-6939
Website: www.emscmn.org

Emergency Nurses Association (ENA)
930 E. Woodfield Rd.
Schaumburg, IL 60173
Toll-Free: 800-900-9659
Phone: 847-460-4000
Website: www.ena.org
E-mail: contact@ena.org

Federal Highway Administration (FHWA)
U.S. Department of Transportation (DOT)
1200 New Jersey Ave. S.E.
Washington, DC 20590
Phone: 202-366-4000
Website: www.fhwa.dot.gov

International Society for Traumatic Stress Studies (ISTSS)

One Parkview Plaza
Ste. 800
Oakbrook Terrace, IL 60181
Phone: 847-686-2234
Fax: 847-686-2251
Website: www.istss.org
E-mail: info@istss.org

King County Emergency Medical Services (EMS)

401 Fifth Ave.
Ste. 1200
Seattle, WA 98104
Phone: 206-296-4693
Fax: 206-296-4866
Website: www.kingcounty.gov/depts/health/emergency-medical-services.aspx

National Association of Emergency Medical Technicians (NAEMT)

P.O. Box 1400
Clinton, MS 39060-1400
Toll-Free: 800-34-NAEMT (800-346-2368)
Phone: 601-924-7744
Fax: 601-924-7325
Website: www.naemt.org
E-mail: info@naemt.org

National Association of EMS Physicians (NAEMSP)

4400 College Blvd.
Ste. 220
Overland Park, KS 66211
Toll-Free: 800-228-3677
Phone: 913-222-8654
Fax: 913-222-8606
Website: www.naemsp.org
E-mail: info-NAEMSP@NAEMSP.org

National EMS Information System (NEMSIS)

P.O. Box 581289
Salt Lake City, UT 84158-1299
Phone: 801-213-3930
Website: www.nemsis.org
E-mail: nemsis@hsc.utah.edu

National Fire Protection Association (NFPA)

1 Batterymarch Park
Massachusetts, MA 02169-7471
Phone: 617-770-3000
Fax: 508-895-8301
Website: www.nfpa.org

National Highway Traffic Safety Administration (NHTSA)

1200 New Jersey Ave. S.E.
W. Bldg.
Washington, DC 20590
Toll-Free: 888-327-4236
Toll-Free TTY: 800-424-9153
Website: www.nhtsa.gov

National Institute of General Medical Sciences (NIGMS)

45 Center Dr.
MSC 6200
Bethesda, MD 20892-6200
Phone: 301-496-7301
Website: nigms.nih.gov
E-mail: info@nigms.nih.gov

National Institute of Neurological Disorders and Stroke (NINDS)

P.O. Box 5801
Bethesda, MD 20824
Toll-Free: 800-352-9424
TTY Relay: 711
Fax: 301-402-2186
Website: www.ninds.nih.gov
E-mail: braininfo@ninds.nih.gov

National Safety Council (NSC)

1121 Spring Lake Dr.
Itasca, IL 60143-3201
Toll-Free: 800-621-7615
Phone: 630-285-1121
Fax: 630-285-1434
Website: www.nsc.org
E-mail: customerservice@nsc.org

National Women's Health Information Center (NWHIC)

Office on Women's Health (OWH)
200 Independence Ave. S.W.
Rm. 712E
Washington, DC 20201
Toll-Free: 800-994-9662
Phone: 202-690-7650
Fax: 202-205-2631
Website: www.womenshealth.gov

Office of Emergency Medical Services (EMS)

National Highway Traffic Safety Administration (NHTSA)
1200 New Jersey Ave. S.E.
Washington, DC 20590
Phone: 202-366-5440
Fax: 202-366-7149
Website: www.ems.gov
E-mail: nhtsa.ems@dot.gov

Shriners International

2900 Rocky Pt. Dr.
Tampa, FL 33607
Phone: 813-281-0300
Website: www.shrinersinternational.org

Society for Academic Emergency Medicine (SAEM)

1111 E. Touhy Ave., Ste. 540
Des Plaines, IL 60018
Phone: 847-813-9823
Fax: 847-813-5450
Website: www.saem.org
E-mail: saem@saem.org

Society of Critical Care Medicine (SCCM)

500 Midway Dr.
Mount Prospect, IL 60056
Phone: 847-827-6888
Fax: 847-439-7226
Website: www.sccm.org
E-mail: support@sccm.org

ThinkFirst

National Injury Prevention Foundation
1801 N. Mill St.
Ste. F
Naperville, IL 60563
Toll-Free: 800-THINK-56 (800-844-6556)
Phone: 630-961-1400
Fax: 630-393-1402
Website: www.thinkfirst.org
E-mail: thinkfirst@thinkfirst.org

U.S. Department of Health and Human Services (HHS)

200 Independence Ave. S.W.
Washington, DC 20201
Toll-Free: 877-696-6775
Website: www.hhs.gov

U.S. Fire Administration (USFA)

16825 S. Seton Ave.
Emmitsburg, MD 21727
Phone: 301-447-1000
Fax: 301-447-1441
Website: www.usfa.fema.gov
E-mail: usfaweb@fema.gov

Chapter 64

Resources for More Information about Disaster Preparedness

American Association of Poison Control Centers (AAPCC)
515 King St.
Ste. 510
Alexandria, VA 22314
Toll-Free: 800-222-1222
Website: www.aapcc.org

American Red Cross
National Headquarters
431 18th St. N.W.
Washington, DC 20006
Toll-Free: 800-REDCROSS (800-733-2767)
Phone: 202-303-4498
Website: www.redcross.org

Boy Scouts of America (BSA)
Emergency Preparedness Plan
P.O. Box 152079
Irving, TX 75015-2079
Phone: 972-580-2000
Website: www.scouting.org

About This Chapter: Resources in this chapter were compiled from several sources deemed reliable; all contact information was verified and updated in July 2019.

Emergency Planning and Community Right-to-Know Act (EPCRA) Hotline

U.S. Environmental Protection Agency (EPA)
1200 Pennsylvania Ave. N.W.
MC 5104A
Washington, DC 20460
Toll-Free: 800-424-9346
Phone: 703-348-5070
Website: www.epa.gov/epcra

Emergency Preparedness and Response

Centers for Disease Control and Prevention (CDC)
1600 Clifton Rd.
Atlanta, GA 30333
Toll-Free: 800-CDC-INFO (800-232-4636)
Website: www.emergency.cdc.gov

Federal Emergency Management Agency (FEMA)

500 C St. S.W.
Washington, DC 20472
Toll-Free: 800-621-FEMA (800-621-3362)
Phone: 202-566-1600
Website: www.fema.gov

Global Disaster Preparedness Center (GDPC)

American Red Cross
431 18th St. N.W.
Washington, DC 20006
Website: www.preparecenter.org
E-mail: gdpc@redcross.org

National Fire Protection Association (NFPA)

Phone: 617-770-3000
Fax: 508-895-8301
Website: www.nfpa.org

National Pesticide Information Center (NPIC)

Oregon State University (OSU)
310 Weniger Hall
Corvallis, OR 97331-6502
Toll-Free: 800-858-7378
Website: www.npic.orst.edu
E-mail: npic@ace.orst.edu

National Safety Council (NSC)

1121 Spring Lake Dr.
Itasca, IL 60143-3201
Phone: 630-285-1121
Fax: 630-285-1315
Website: www.nsc.org
E-mail: info@nsc.org

Office of Air Quality Planning and Standards (OAQPS)

MD C404-03
Research Triangle Park, NC 27711
Phone: 919-541-5504
Website: www3.epa.gov/airquality/contact.html

Safe Drinking Water Hotline

U.S. Environmental Protection Agency (EPA)
1200 Pennsylvania Ave. N.W.
MC 4606M
Washington, DC 20460
Toll-Free: 888-395-1033
Website: www.epa.gov/ground-water-and-drinking-water/safe-drinking-water-information

STORET Water Quality System Hotline

U.S. Environmental Protection Agency (EPA)
1200 Pennsylvania Ave. N.W.
Washington, DC 20460
Toll-Free: 800-424-9067
Website: www.epa.gov/storet
E-mail: STORET@epa.gov

U.S. Department of Homeland Security (DHS)

Phone: 202-282-8000
Website: www.dhs.gov

U.S. Environmental Protection Agency (EPA)

Clean Air Markets Division
1200 Pennsylvania Ave. N.W.
MC 6204M
Washington, DC 20460
Phone: 202-343-9620
Website: www.epa.gov

U.S. Fire Administration (USFA)

16825 S. Seton Ave.
Emmitsburg, MD 21727
Phone: 301-447-1000
Fax: 301-447-1441
Website: www.usfa.fema.gov
E-mail: usfaweb@fema.gov

Index

Index

Page numbers that appear in *Italics* refer to tables or illustrations. Page numbers that have a small 'n' after the page number refer to citation information shown as Notes. Page numbers that appear in **Bold** refer to information contained in boxes within the chapters.

A

AAFP *see* American Academy of Family Physicians
abdominal thrusts, choking 101
abuse *see* sexual abuse
accident
    coping with a traumatic experience 41
    fractures 67
    statistics 7
    see also car accident
ACEP *see* American College of Emergency Physicians
addiction, opioids 109
aggressive driving
    overview 181–3
    safety savvy 210
    speeding 186
"Aggressive Driving" (Omnigraphics) 181n
aggressive skates, skating 287
Agricultural Research Service (ARS)
    publication
        first aid basics 25n
airbags
    overview 133–9
    safety belts 130
    spinal cord injury (SCI) **77**
"Air Bags" (NHTSA) 133n

alarm
    carbon monoxide 237
    fire safety 222
alcohol
    defensive driving 120
    drugged driving 178
    impaired driving 171
    motorcycle safety 195
    night driving 154
    pedestrian safety 198
    poison prevention tips 247
    safety savvy 206
    teen drivers 116
    winter storms 327
alcohol overdose, overview 105–8
alcoholic beverages, poison prevention tips 247
all-terrain vehicles (ATVs)
    overview 281–3
    tire safety 141
    traumatic brain injury (TBI) 95
"All-Terrain Vehicles and Work" (CDC) 281n
allergies
    alcohol overdose 107
    insect stings 55
    poison prevention tips 245
alprazolam (Xanax), alcohol overdose 106
Ambien (zolpidem), alcohol overdose 106

M

N

X

Y

Z